# Intermittent Fasting

*Reset your Metabolism with The Ketogenic Diet, Burn Fat Through Meal Plan, Low Carb, Combined With The Powerful Intermittent Fasting Method*

**Kathleen Ashley**

Regardless, there are zero scenarios where the original author or the Publisher can be deemed liable in any fashion for any damages or hardships that may result from any of the information discussed herein.

Additionally, the information in the following pages is intended only for informational purposes and should thus be thought of as universal. As befitting its nature, it is presented without assurance regarding its prolonged validity or interim quality. Trademarks that are mentioned are done without written consent and can in no way be considered an endorsement from the trademark holder.

# Table of Contents

# Introduction

Congratulations on downloading *Intermittent Fasting* and thank you for doing so.

The following chapters will discuss the keto diet and intermittent fasting. It is important to have a good understanding of the history and the mechanics of the keto diet and intermittent fasting before embarking on a practice of either. We will explore a brief history of each, learning where and how both began and how these methods can be used to improve your overall weight loss results. By individually exploring the mechanics and benefits of each method, learning how the two systems work well together, what is involved to fully use them to your advantage, and the benefits to your overall health, you will have a better understanding of these methods and their role in your personal health and well-being. In this book, there will be suggestions for lifestyle changes, meal plans, and the role of exercising, all designed to make this new behavior a part of your everyday routine with minimum effort. We understand that no plan will work for you if you do not understand it completely or if the execution of those plans does not fit well into your current lifestyle. We will also discuss which foods are best for inclusion in the keto diet, and which foods you should leave at the grocery store. Once you understand all the mechanics of the keto diet and intermittent fasting, you will be well prepared to embark on your new journey and start changing your life.

There are plenty of books on this subject on the market, so thanks again for choosing this one! Every effort was made to ensure it is full of as much useful information as possible. Please enjoy!

# Chapter 1: A History of Intermittent Fasting and the Keto Diet

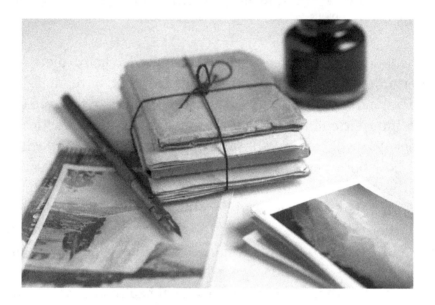

Fasting is the act of voluntarily refusing food intake for many various reasons. Fasting has been used since ancient times as a part of spiritual celebrations and for health reasons. Why would we choose to voluntarily give up eating food? The idea behind performing a sacrifice is to give up something of great personal value to cause personal suffering to put oneself closer to one's goal. Few things are filled with greater personal value to us than our next meal. Whether a person's particular goal is spiritual enlightenment or better health, food is often very difficult for most people to do without, therefore giving the act of fasting the potential to become a great personal struggle.

Fasting involves the complete avoidance from food, drink, or both. This can be done for religious or health-related reasons. Sometimes fasting is used in observance of a ritual. Sometimes fasting is used to protest certain behaviors. The period one sets as a period of fasting may be complete or partial, of a long or a short time period, or intermittent. Fasting has been practiced and promoted since the dawn of time all over the world. Doctors have long recommended it for the care and treatment of certain conditions. Founders and followers of many religions use fasting as part of their religious rituals and celebrations. Many religions have set days or time periods when almost all followers are required to fast. Sometimes fasting is used by groups and individuals as part of the initiation rites for club membership. And, since the dawn of time, different individuals and groups have used fasting as a way to cleanse the body and the soul and to prepare oneself for the coming of their deity. Fasting has also been used to protest the poor treatment of other people or to show solidarity and agreement with a particular group or idea. Fasting is ultimately a powerful tool. As long as the person is conscious and has control of their faculties, no one can force them to consume food.

The Greek physician Hippocrates is believed to be the first one in history to use fasting for therapeutic reasons. His uses and experiments began as early as the fifth century BCE.

He recommended fasting to patients who showed signs of certain illnesses. Hippocrates probably felt that fasting would be a natural cure for combating certain symptoms. He most likely noticed that many people who were feeling ill simply lost their appetites for food and drink and still recovered complete health eventually. Many doctors still believe that administering food or drink during such states was unnecessary and possibly even detrimental. This certainly holds true even today with some illnesses. Anytime you have a virus that affects the digestive tract you are advised to refrain from solid food and take only liquids as soon as your stomach can tolerate them. This was and is true because fasting has been shown to be an important natural part of the recovery process.

A better understanding of the effects of fasting on the human body began to evolve in the latter part of the 19th century. This was a time when some of the first organized studies of fasting, which included abstinence from both food and drink, were begun to be carried out as controlled experiments in humans and animals. Moving into the beginning of the twentieth century more became known about the nutritional requirements of the human body. Scientists and physicians were better able to know what foods were best for overall good nutrition and what foods should be given to people who were ill or suffered from certain conditions. Different methods of fasting became ever more sophisticated, and during this time a wide variety of fasting plans were experimented with. During this time, more physicians began using fasting as a form of treatment of certain diseases. Fasting was also used as a form of disease prevention for certain diseases. The study and implementation of fasting were carried out in different and varied locations. It became very popular in hospitals and clinics, and even some use at home was begun under the supervision of the family doctor. Fasting methods applied for the treatment of certain diseases could be prescribed to last for more than a month. These plans allowed the patient to consume only water or plain coffee or tea and always included gentle exercise and the use of enemas. Methods known as modified fasting allowed for the patient to consume no more than two hundred to five hundred calories daily. Calories were generally consumed in the form of milk, honey, bone broth, fruit juice, vegetable broth, and bread. Spiritual and psychological therapies were often included to allow the patient to receive a full range of physical and mental treatment. Many physicians began using diets as low as eight hundred calories as weight loss methods for obese people.

They would then alternate periods of eating with periods of

fasting to facilitate even faster weight loss. This is when the use of intermittent fasting really began to become popular. This type of fasting involved specified periods of calorie consumption followed by specified periods of calorie restriction, thus the term 'intermittent.'

Although fasting was clearly documented as the best choice of treatment for certain diseases, particularly when that disease was naturally accompanied by a loss of appetite, by the beginning of the twenty-first century there still was not a lot of research documented as to whether fasting would be the treatment of choice for all diseases or any other known human condition. As an example, intermittent fasting and its benefits had long been studied in humans with symptoms of diabetes. This research suggested that intermittent fasting, when adhered to strictly for a period of at least fifteen days, was known to improve the effects of glucose absorption by the human body that had previously only been treatable by insulin. Comparable studies carried out in laboratories using rodents showed much the same results. Scientists found that long term fasting by the rodents promoted their bodies to no longer tolerate a large intake of glucose and also prompted the release of body toxins from the rodent's tissues.

Fasting was long practiced by people and civilizations during religious preparations. Priests and priestesses especially used fasting as a way to prepare for the approach of religious deities. Many cultures practice fasting to make peace with a god they believe they have angered, or to resurrect a god believed to have died. Today fasting is still observed for special reasons and before or during sacred times and other times of religious celebration. And besides its role in religious celebrations, many religious and political figures have used fasting as a means to promote and call attention to social unrest or injustice.

Intermittent fasting can easily be thought of as a long-ignored secret to facilitating improved health. It was developed by people in cultures we only read about in history books. Humans have been practicing fasting at different times and for different reasons throughout all of human history. But why do we think of it as a secret? We think of it as a secret because this powerful weapon designed to improve overall health has become mostly relegated to the pages of dusty medical books and historical and religious writings.

But fasting is a powerful dietary tool that, when used properly, carries huge bonuses for the overall improvement of human health. Fasting can still be used to assist in the care and treatment of many human conditions, such as the treatment of Type 2 Diabetes. It is proven to aid in weight loss by limiting the time periods when we are allowed to take in food. People who fast regularly will soon notice a dramatic increase in their energy levels. They will find they are able to participate in more physical activities for longer time periods. And an added bonus is the potential to save a lot of money and time. You can expect to save time and money in several ways:

- Buying less junk food
- Eating less overall
- Less illness due to improved health
- Better efficiency due to improved overall feeling of health
- Less days missing work
- Less money spent buying medications to cure illnesses

Besides the above-mentioned reasons, throughout history, humans have often fasted for reasons beyond their control. There have been many instances where food simply was not available. Whether it was pioneers traveling across country or an area-wide crop failure, if food was not available through farming or hunting, people did without. They fasted. This is not the type of fasting we will concentrate on. We are interested in voluntary, choice-driven fasting.

In recent years intermittent fasting has become a new and exciting way of life for many people. Whether they use it for weight loss, to improve overall health, or to lessen the effects of a disease, intermittent fasting can be used for many different reasons and in many different ways. And the term 'intermittent' implies that the fasting period is whatever and whenever you decide it to be, and that it is totally within your control to start or stop as you see necessary.

There is one important difference between fasting and starvation. That difference is personal control. Starvation implies that there is no food to eat. You would eat if food were offered, but there is none to offer you. Starvation is not done on purpose, and it usually can't be controlled. Fasting is done on purpose. Fasting is done voluntarily. Fasting is done with the knowledge of risks and benefits, and how the benefits greatly outweigh the risks for the majority of people who fast. Fasting means you purposely deny yourself the consumption of food to reach some greater gain, like physical health or spiritual growth.

You can fast for any prescribed period of time. The duration of the fast is totally up to you. You can fast for a few hours, a few days, or a few weeks. You are in charge of how long the fast will last. Fasting has no set time period that you do not make yourself. Since fasting is nothing more than the absence of eating, you can end your fast any time you chose. If you are not eating, then you are fasting.

The keto diet actually became popular in the 1920s. It was developed and used as a way to treat epilepsy. Doctors discovered that the strict food choices of the keto diet offered the patient relief from seizures. It also offered an alternative choice to the fasting method which had previously been used effectively in the treatment of seizures although scientists did not know why at the time, there was apparently a link between the withholding of food and the cessation of seizures.

As early as 1911 scientists were doing research into ways to cure epilepsy or, in the absence of a cure, to allow the patient some relief from the seizures that sometimes made normal everyday activities impossible tasks.

At that time, the treatment of choice for epilepsy was potassium bromide. Unfortunately, this chemical, while it did help with the seizures, had a profoundly negative effect of patient's mental capacities by causing diminished cognitive function. So one scientist began a study where twenty patients with epilepsy followed a low-calorie, totally vegetarian food plan combined with intermittent fasting. Two of the twenty patients actually showed marked improvement in their symptoms. Most of the patients were unable to follow the strict dietary restrictions long enough to see if the diet would be effective. The diet was found to be preferable to the negative side effects of the potassium bromide.

But while this strict vegetarian diet provided relief to the patient, not eating was not seen as a viable way to live. People need food to be able to grow and develop; to be able to work and function in the world. Experimentation with different foods began, and the keto diet was born.

The diet became less favorable when medication was developed that could limit or eliminate seizures in most people. It was far more convenient to take a pill or an injection and be able to eat and drink as other people did. Also, the diet was inconvenient for other reasons. Treatment usually began with a period of total fasting lasting up to a month, during which time the patient only consumed water. This treatment was believed to release the toxins from the body that caused the seizures. After this prolonged fasting, specific food was reintroduced in small amounts.

It was not known exactly why this method worked until many years later when science had developed to the point where instruments and tests could study the results of certain actions on the human body. It was eventually discovered that, during periods of starvation, the liver released three specific enzymes that worked together to suppress certain functions in the body, like epileptic seizures. Scientists were excited to study just what other diseases could be suppressed or eradicated by using either fasting or the keto diet, or a combination of the two. This was discovered in the early 1960s and quickly created a renewed interest in the study and usefulness of fasting and the keto diet.

In the early 1970s, researchers developed a keto diet that included the use of fats, oils, and so-called 'good' carbohydrates to enable people to create more varied and interesting meals. During the body-conscious eras of the 1970s and 1980s, the Atkins diet came to the forefront of American culture. Dr. Robert Atkins created it and offered a modification on the strict keto diet by allowing more carbohydrate intake. The benefit of the keto diet over the Atkins diet is its strict diet plan and adherence to the formula, making it less likely to fail if followed properly.

The keto diet is strict, but that is exactly the program many people need to enable them to succeed in their weight loss goals. If your current way of eating was working, you wouldn't be looking for an alternative! The strictness of the keto diet, rigidly following the food suggestions and dietary restrictions will give you the greatest level of success in your new endeavor toward a healthier you. Adding in intermittent fasting will give you another level of control over your diet and well-being: the choice to eat when you choose to eat.

By combining intermittent fasting and the keto diet, you have the tools needed to take you to a new and improved level of health and happiness.

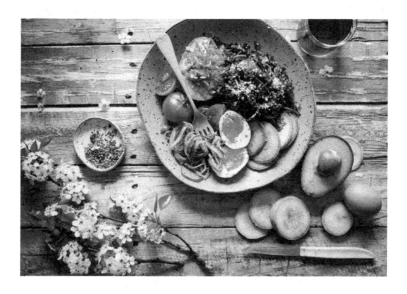

Your new journey may not be easy, but it will definitely be beneficial in the long run. You will make mistakes; everyone does. You might become frustrated, especially in the beginning. Do not give up! There are variations to the keto diet and to intermittent fasting that can be paired in any number of combinations to enable you to be the best you possible.

# Chapter 2: What Is Intermittent Fasting and How Does It Benefit Your Health

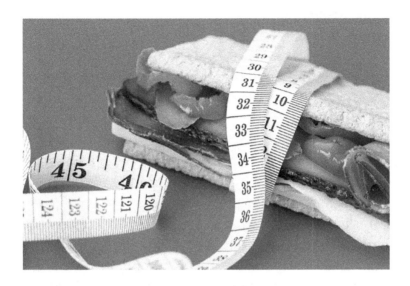

So what exactly is intermittent fasting? It is exactly what it says it is—fasting on an intermittent, non-continuous basis. It is the conscious act of planning exactly when you will eat and when you will not eat. It is the act of taking control of exactly when you will intake food and when you will refrain from eating. It gives you the power to decide, and that power is often lacking in many dietary plans. The feeling of having control over your habits is just another way to make you feel stronger in your choice to move toward healthier habits.

Fasting is the most basic of functions that will allow the human body to burn off toxins and look to itself for fuel and energy. Without food coming in, the body will look to its own stores for fat to burn. This is actually a very normal state for the body to be in; actually, the body was made to do this. In times of famine, the body naturally turns to itself and the excess fat it has stored away to be able to maintain life while searching for a new food source. Your body fat is nothing more than food that your body has stored away for you to use when needed. We were genetically designed to do this. It's just been in recent years that lifestyle choices have caused many people to store away much more fat than they really need.

The best way to describe intermittent fasting is to think of it as a constant cycle between eating and not eating. No method or style of fasting will ever tell you which foods you should or should not eat or which diet plan is best to follow. Intermittent fasting only pertains to the specific time periods in which you do or do not eat. Intermittent fasting should never be thought of as a diet, especially not the average description of a diet, but rather it is a pattern of eating at precise times. There are several common patterns to intermittent fasting. Historically our ancestors faced everyday life without shopping at the grocery store or raiding the fridge during a midnight raid. Food was not always available for the taking. At many times there was nothing available to eat. Because of these forced periods of food deprivation, our ancestors slowly evolved into human beings who were able to carry on their daily activities without the benefit of regular meals for long periods of time. As a matter of fact, the practice of fasting periodically is a much more normal state for humans than to be constantly eating.

Fasting is not some scary ancient tradition. It can definitely be used as a normal part of everyday life. Viewed as a tool for dietary reasons, it is probably the oldest and strongest we have available. Over the years, humans seem to have forgotten the enormous power of this simple tool. Once we have learned all the tools that go into a proper fast, we have the ability to use fasting to our advantage.

Losing weight allows the body to restore balance to its internal systems. There is no magic formula when it comes to losing weight. To be successful, we only need to increase the length of time we use to let our bodies burn food for energy. We call this intermittent fasting. Simply speaking, stored energy is used for fuel when we chose to fast. That is the precise reason the body has stored the fat. Many people are confused by the idea that it is good for the body to do without food. Many people feel that abstaining from food will lead to starvation. That is possible if food is never eaten. But with intermittent fasting, we simply refrain from eating food for a specific period of time to allow our bodies to snack on its own food stores. Our bodies were built to do this. Mammals do this. That is how the human body is designed to operate.

Eating constantly never allows the body to burn stored fat for fuel and energy. The body will continue to rely on the steady stream of incoming food to take care of its needs. You will never lose excess body fat. You will keep it stored away. The body will assume that we are storing food to prepare for an upcoming period of famine. When you do this, your body lacks balance. When you do this, your lifestyle will never improve.

Voluntarily deciding to give up eating food for a certain number of hours each day or a certain number of days each week provides multiple benefits to both your brain and your body. We have evolved to take advantage of fasting. People did not have access to unlimited snacks and three-square meals each day until the most modern of times. Evolution took humans through time periods when there was not much food available if any at all. Our bodies have learned to thrive during intermittent fasting. Gathering food today is much easier when we can just make a short trip to the grocery store or swing through the nearest fast food drive-thru. Our new sedentary life is not very helpful either. Now that many jobs are done sitting down, not requiring any form of physical exertion, and we have the ability to eat as much as we want whenever we want, it is no wonder so many people are looking for a way to reverse the effects this lifestyle is causing. Our bodies were never meant to be treated this way.

Intermittent fasting can definitely help you leave the diet yo-yo behind, even if it is something you have been struggling with for the bulk of your life, as many of us have. You need to be prepared to make intermittent fasting a standard part of your overall lifestyle. The number one problem most people have with the idea of intermittent fasting is in being able to make the practice fit into everyday life. We have jobs, families, commitments; we have a life to take care of. And intermittent fasting is only one piece of the lifestyle change puzzle.

Intermittent fasting is not a diet. It is the conscious choice of a lifestyle that allows you to decide the specific times of day and the specific days when you will eat.

It is also possible to choose to fast on specific days, or for periods of days, rather than daily for a specific time. You can consume only water during this time or use a mixture of water-based drinks such as plain black coffee and plain tea. These are allowed because they contain no protein, sugars, or carbohydrates. If you keep these three items out of your diet, your body remains in the fasting state. As long as the body remains in the fasting state, it will continue to turn to itself to raid stored fat for energy. And this is exactly why intermittent fasting is the preferred choice for maximum weight loss. With fasting, the first few hours and days offer the biggest return on investment; you will burn the most fat in the first forty-eight hours. After that, the efficiency of the fat burning begins to slow down. The body, in a prolonged time of food being withheld, begins to assume that this will be a long-term starvation due to the lack of food. It will begin to slow the rate at which it digs into fat stores to allow those stores to last longer. The body feels a little food at a time is better than running out of food stores too soon.

Eating is the act of putting food into our bodies to use later as fuel. Eating is a pleasurable social act that we can share with family and friends. Unfortunately, sometimes we overindulge in this pleasure and find ourselves carrying around extra pounds in the form of stored fat. We do need regular food intake to fuel the body and give us enough energy to carry out our daily activities. The human body quite regularly stores excess food for fuel to burn later. If the body was not able to store some food for fat the humans would be forced to constantly take in food; to remain in a constantly fed state. The key to the storage of fat from food is a hormone called insulin. The human body creates insulin in response to food intake. Insulin has two different ways to help the body store fat. The body uses insulin to link sugars gathered from foods into glycogen that is then stored in the liver for future use. Unfortunately, or maybe fortunately for us, the liver is a small organ with limited storage space.

Once the storage space in the liver is full, the body then begins turning the excess sugar into fat and storing it in various places throughout the body. This is a more complicated process, but it builds up over time. There is absolutely no limit to the space that the body can find to store fat in secret places. When all the available space is full, the body just adds on the already stored fat by displacing internal organs and stretching the skin to make the fat fit inside.

The process begins to work in reverse when we chose not to eat and instead take advantage of intermittent fasting. Since food is not being consumed insulin is not being produced. This lack of insulin tells the body it is time to begin burning fat stores for energy since it is not currently able to get more energy from consumed food. Blood sugar levels begin to fall throughout the fast. The body must now pull from fat stores for energy. It turns to the liver and its stores of glycogen first. Glycogen is the body's most readily available source of energy, in the event that food consumption is not an option. The body takes the glycogen from the liver and breaks it down into glucose molecules to use for energy and fuel by all the systems of the body. The amount of glycogen stored in the liver can provide up to forty-eight hours of energy for the cells of the body. Once the supply of glycogen is used up the body will turn to stored fat for more energy. And that is the goal of intermittent fasting: to cause the body to get to a state where it uses fat stores for energy and fuel, thus eliminating these fat stores and leading to a healthier you.

Diets can be complicated. Sometimes dieting takes over your life, ruling where you will be able to go and what you will be able to eat, drink, do. Fasting works to simplify life by removing the driving need to constantly eat. Some diets are very expensive to follow properly. Fasting, on the other hand, is absolutely free. It costs you nothing to do without food! And fasting can be done anytime or anywhere, unlike many diets that require complicated equipment or following complicated recipes. The diet you chose may or may not work for you, but fasting will provide marvelous health benefits to almost everyone. Very few people are unable to take advantage of intermittent fasting. And it is a viable way to improve your overall health without the use of medications.

There are several methods of intermittent fasting. The key to your success will be in choosing the fasting plan that best fits your lifestyle. Some of the most popular ones that we will explore are the eat-stop-eat method, the 16:8 method, and the 5:2 method of fasting.

The eat-stop-eat method is just what it sounds like; you eat, you stop, then you eat again. The following chart shows an example of how to set a schedule for this particular type of intermittent fasting.

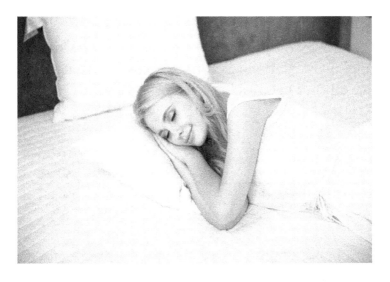

| | SUN | MON | TUES | WEDS | THURS | FRI | SAT |
|---|---|---|---|---|---|---|---|
| MIDNIGHT | SLEEPS | SLEEPS | SLEEPS | SLEEPS | SLEEPS | SLEEPS | SLEEPS |
| 4:00 AM | SLEEPS | SLEEPS | SLEEPS | SLEEPS | SLEEPS | SLEEPS | SLEEPS |
| 8:00 AM | SLEEPS | SLEEPS | SLEEPS | SLEEPS | SLEEPS | SLEEPS | SLEEPS |
| NOON | EATING | FASTING | EATING | FASTING | EATING | FASTING | EATING |
| 4:00 PM | EATING | FASTING | EATING | FASTING | EATING | FASTING | EATING |
| 8:00 PM | EATING | FASTING | EATING | FASTING | EATING | FASTING | EATING |
| MIDNIGHT | SLEEPS | SLEEPS | SLEEPS | SLEEPS | SLEEPS | SLEEPS | SLEEPS |

As shown in the preceding table, certain days are set aside for fasting. On the days that fasting is scheduled, if you are not sleeping, you will not eat. It is recommended to fast two to three days per week. You may, of course, fast longer than the chart indicates if you feel comfortable with it. In the beginning, it is recommended to keep your schedule to a one day fast until your body adjusts to the regular absence of food. Also, remember that fasting means no food intake is allowed. You must remember to keep yourself well hydrated with water or plain tea or coffee. Keto friendly Bulletproof coffee is also an option. You have the freedom to choose how many days you will fast.

With the 16:8 method of intermittent fasting, as is shown in the following chart, you will fast for sixteen hours each day and consume all your calories in eight hours each day.

|  | SUN | MON | TUES | WED | THURS | FRI | SAT |
|---|---|---|---|---|---|---|---|
| MIDNIGHT | SLEEPS | SLEEPS | SLEEPS | SLEEPS | SLEEPS | SLEEPS | SLEEPS |
| 4:00 AM | SLEEPS | SLEEPS | SLEEPS | SLEEPS | SLEEPS | SLEEPS | SLEEPS |
| 8:00 AM | SLEEPS | SLEEPS | SLEEPS | SLEEPS | SLEEPS | SLEEPS | SLEEPS |
| NOON | EATING | EATING | EATING | EATING | EATING | EATING | EATING |
| 4:00 PM | EATING | EATING | EATING | EATING | EATING | EATING | EATING |
| 8:00 PM | EATING | EATING | EATING | EATING | EATING | EATING | EATING |
| MIDNIGHT | SLEEPS | SLEEPS | SLEEPS | SLEEPS | SLEEPS | SLEEPS | SLEEPS |

Whether all your calories are consumed in one, two, or three meals; or one meal and one light snack, or several light snacks, does not matter. The most important point is that all calories are consumed in the eight-hour window ONLY. The remainder of the day is set aside for fasting. You may not necessarily be asleep during the entire time, but if you schedule your fasting period to coincide with your sleeping period, you have a natural excuse not to eat. Since most people average between seven and nine hours of sleep each night, this covers a large chunk of the time you are required to be food free. During the few hours, you are awake and fasting just remember to stay well hydrated by sipping water or black coffee or plain tea. This is also a good time to enjoy a cup of keto friendly Bulletproof coffee.

The 5:2 method of fasting is similar to the 16:8 method of fasting in that it sets aside specific times for fasting, as the chart below shows us.

|  | SUN | MON | TUES | WEDS | THURS | FRI | SAT |
|---|---|---|---|---|---|---|---|
| MIDNIGHT | SLEEPS | SLEEPS | SLEEPS | SLEEPS | SLEEPS | SLEEPS | SLEEPS |
| 4:00 AM | SLEEPS | SLEEPS | SLEEPS | SLEEPS | SLEEPS | SLEEPS | SLEEPS |
| 8:00 AM | SLEEPS | SLEEPS | SLEEPS | SLEEPS | SLEEPS | SLEEPS | SLEEPS |
| NOON | EATING | FASTING | EATING | EATING | FASTING | EATING | EATING |
| 4:00 PM | EATING | FASTING | EATING | EATING | FASTING | EATING | EATING |
| 8:00 PM | EATING | FASTING | EATING | EATING | FASTING | EATING | EATING |
| MIDNIGHT | SLEEPS | SLEEPS | SLEEPS | SLEEPS | SLEEPS | SLEEPS | SLEEPS |

This method is similar in structure to the 16:8 method, where certain days are set aside for fasting. However, with this method the fast days can be periods of total fasting or they can be periods of restricted calories, usually no more than five hundred to six hundred calories consumed. During the times of fasting if you are not actually eating food then remember to stay well hydrated with water or plain tea or black coffee. A nice cup of keto friendly Bulletproof coffee.

The most important feature of the fasting schedule is that it can be adjusted to fit your particular scheduling needs. Do you work from home? The times for eating can be adjusted to later in the day, as long as they coincide with the hours you are awake so that you are free to enjoy a family meal at the end of the day. Do you work second or third shift? Just as your day might be 'backwards' from the normal nine to five working day, the eating/fasting schedule can be adjusted to fit into your overnight hours. Do you work manual labor Monday through

Friday and sleep all weekend, rebuilding stamina for the next work week? Those days of rest can be your fasting days since you won't be expending the usual amount of energy requiring food intake. The important thing to note is that the fasting schedule can be worked into any work/life schedule. You will fast when it is convenient for you. Just remember to fast mainly when asleep.

One thing that keeps many people from beginning a program of regular intermittent fasting is the fear of hunger. We, humans, worry about hunger. Sometimes we even fear to be hungry. We do not want to be hungry. We fear hunger because it means there is no food and then we will starve and then we will probably die. I promise you this will not happen when you are using a controlled fast like intermittent fasting. Remember, as long as the fasting is done for a set period of time, then hunger that you feel in the beginning is a temporary thing. It comes and goes, in waves that rise and fall within the body. It will not become an unbearable monster that drives you to eat everything in the kitchen. If you feel hunger while fasting, get busy doing something. If the hunger does not soon pass, as it should, then sip a cup of black coffee or a glass of unsweetened tea. This will help ease the hunger pangs.

So what can intermittent fasting mean to you? Well, intermittent fasting has many proven health benefits. The single most important reason people give for fasting, besides religious reasons, is to aid in weight loss. Taking in fewer calories than the body needs is the first step in weight loss. When you begin to lose weight, the body can experience other important changes with very little effort. As weight decreases so do blood sugar levels and cholesterol levels, since these are driven by food intake and body weight. Lower sugar levels mean lower insulin levels. Insulin is the chemical the pancreas puts out to counteract sugar in the bloodstream. Higher levels of sugar mean higher levels of insulin, and insulin in the bloodstream is a major contributor to fat storage. This phenomenon is what aids in the reversal of Type 2 Diabetes, which is purely driven by excess body weight and poor dietary choices. As your total weight decreases the joints in the lower body may begin to feel better since excess body weight causes increased strain on the knees and hips. In fact, one pound of excess weight adds four pounds of pressure to a knee joint. Also, weight loss brings an overall increased sense of wellbeing. It's difficult to feel good when excess pounds are causing you to feel sluggish, and with this comes increased mental clarity and concentration and better thinking and decision-making abilities.

Done correctly, the benefits of intermittent fasting far outweigh any negative effects that might come from missing a few meals. In fact, there really are no negative effects from fasting if it is done properly. We, humans, were meant to miss meals and cleanse our bodies on a regular basis. Our bodies were never meant to store great globs of excess fat under our skin and around our internal organs in case we might need it at some later date. You might feel some hunger in the beginning, but once you adjust to your new fasting schedule, you will quickly see results that will far outweigh any hunger pains you might experience.

# Chapter 3: What Is the Keto Diet and How Does It Benefit Your Health

The ketogenic diet, more commonly known as the keto diet, is a plan where carbohydrate intake is kept low in favor of consuming more proteins and fats. The main goal of following the keto diet plan is to create amazing levels weight loss through intensive fat-burning. The ultimate goal is to lose weight quickly and to eventually make the body feel fuller while suffering from fewer cravings. This diet will cause effects that will result in amazing mood-boosting feelings. Your mental focusing abilities will increase rapidly, and you will experience an amazing upsurge in energy. By slashing the amount of carbohydrates, you consume on a regular basis and instead filling up on good fats and proteins, you will safely enter a state of ketosis. When you enter the state of ketosis your body will begin to break down both dietary fat and stored body fat into substances called ketones. Now your body's fat burning system will rely primarily on fat– instead of sugar – for needed fuel and energy. While this condition is similar to what happens in some popular, commercial low-carb diet plans, the extreme carb restrictions of the keto diet – where you will regularly consume no more than about 20 net carbs a day or less, depending on the version of the diet that you follow – that cause the body to deliberately shift into ketosis. And that is precisely what makes this increasingly popular diet plan the one people are turning to more and more every day to start them on the road to weight loss and good health.

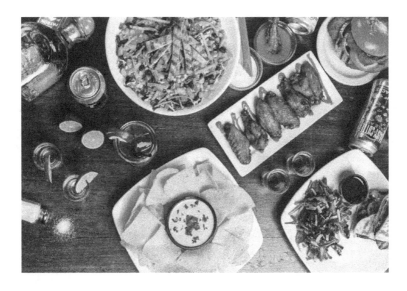

If you have spent any time over the past few years studying diet plans or listening to mainstream conversation, then you have heard of the keto diet. This diet is a low-carbohydrate high-fat eating plan that has become the new darling of pop culture and the world at large. Celebrities love the keto diet. Everyday more and more people delve into the mysteries of the keto diet, wondering if it is the magic bullet that will finally lead them down that glorious path where weight loss meets improved health. Well, unfortunately, no diet plan is a magic bullet, but the keto diet plan is pretty amazing. After reading this book, we hope you will come away with a better understanding of exactly how the keto diet works and exactly how it can help lead you down that path to a better way of life.

In one way of thinking, the ketogenic diet has been a part of man's way of life since they ran around chasing the dinosaurs while searching for food. Agriculture, the practice of growing fruits and vegetables for human consumption, is a fairly recent way of life, other than the small home farms that people maintained for personal use. When we talk about the various ways that humans have used over the years to feed themselves, growing things in the ground was not a prominent part of the early history of man. Early man was a hunter.

Early man hunted meat, traveling from place to place in search of bigger and better game to kill to allow him to feed the family. Most of the areas of the world that humans lived in were simply too cold for any real attempt at growing things to be successful enough to produce enough food to sustain life on a long-term basis. So basically, our ancestors survived for centuries on the protein and fat that they consumed from animals, with the odd bit of fruit or veggie thrown in when they could be found and gathered during hunting trips.

This is just a little illustration to prove a very important point—that the human body was not meant to survive on an overabundance of carbohydrates. Even in areas of the world where carbohydrates in the form of pasta or rice are regularly consumed, the diet also features meats in minimal amounts with larger amounts of fish and vegetables. It is very easy to understand why our bodies respond so well to a ketogenic diet. It is the diet our bodies have adapted to through the process of evolution to be able to live on. Obesity was most likely not a problem for the average cave person who was struggling to find enough food for him and his family to eat. But in current times we do not need to look very far around us to see several morbidly obese people. There seems to be a direct link between the fact that so many people are currently struggling with weight issues and weight loss when the bulk of the normal diet is made up of primarily carbohydrates and sugar.

The keto diet was first developed in the early 1920s. Doctors discovered, through trial and error, that patients who were fed a restrictive diet of high protein, high fats, and low amounts of carbohydrates could reduce or eliminate seizures suffered by people with epilepsy. The doctors and researchers found that this diet helped nearly eighty percent of patients. This diet was especially effective when it was prescribed for children because parents could easily control the types and amounts of food and drink that their children consumed. Doctors continued prescribing this method of treatment for several decades until anti-convulsing drugs were developed. As we moved into a more industrialized type of society, people found it was much easier to take a medication to control or cure their seizures and not be forced to worry about being tied to a strict diet regimen.

So the keto diet plan languished almost completely into obscurity until the mid-1990s. At that time the parents of a young boy were desperately seeking a way to control the devastating seizures that threatened his very way of life. At times his seizures were so bad that he was unable to function normally. Through intensive research, his parents discovered descriptions of the keto diet and its promises of, if not necessarily a cure for their son, a definite reduction in symptoms. With nothing to lose, they began feeding their son a strict keto diet, carefully monitoring every morsel of food the child consumed and when he consumed it. Within just a few days of beginning the diet, his seizures stopped completely. After following the diet for many years, he remains seizure free even as an adult.

Thankfully for its millions of followers, the benefits of the keto diet do not end with treating and curing epilepsy. If the keto diet was only useful for controlling epilepsy, then the masses would not have so eagerly adopted it as their diet of choice. Most people today are far more interested in the potential of the diet to help them with weight loss. No one knows for certain when the keto diet first became popular as a method for losing significant amounts of weight. However, this renewed interest in the keto diet is causing researchers to take a renewed interest in the mechanics and effects of the diet itself.

The keto diet is not just a license to eat all the meat you want to eat as often as you want to eat it. The keto diet is a specifically orchestrated food plan that must be followed as closely as possible in order to achieve maximum results. The diet plan features less dependence on carbohydrates and more dependence on a greater intake of proteins and fats, especially those good fats that are the staple of the keto diet. Yes, there are good fats! When carbohydrate intake is restricted, the body will naturally turn to stored fats for fuel, thus decreasing fat stores which will automatically lead to less body weight. And the end result is weight loss!

The way this process works is simple. By taking in fewer carbohydrates, you will force the body to turn to its own stores of fat for energy and fuel. This is a normal function of the body, a feature designed to keep humans from actually starving to death when food isn't readily available for a short period of time. As the body begins to work on consuming and eliminating fat stores, it creates chemicals called ketones that are used to fuel the body and the brain.

Once the body begins producing ketones on a regular basis a state of ketosis is reached. Ketosis is, in reality, a mild form of ketoacidosis which is actually a side effect of diabetes. Experts are divided on whether or not ketosis is safe for the human body. Ketoacidosis is definitely not safe and requires immediate medical attention. But ketosis is generally seen as a natural side effect of consuming a low carbohydrate diet and a necessary state for the body to reach in order to begin maximum weight loss. Proponents of the keto diet feel that the mild form of ketosis reached is not enough to be harmful if the diet is followed correctly, but a needed state of being to reach in order to reap the full benefits of the diet.

Since the human body can only store about a two-day supply of glucose, in the form of glycogen, generally two or three days of a diet consisting of less than 20 grams of carbohydrates daily is enough time for the body to enter ketosis. Reducing your consumption of carbs on a regular basis is the most important method for pushing the body into ketosis. Once the body has reached a state of ketosis, it will remain in a state of ketosis until the time when you begin to consume more than the keto diet daily recommended amount of carbohydrates. If that happens, the body will come out of ketosis and will once again begin storing excess food sugars as fat. To be able to re-enter a state of ketosis would require dropping the carbohydrate count back down to the recommended dietary levels.

Besides being an effective treatment for epilepsy, what else can a keto diet do for you? Well, the diet has many health advantages. The number one advantage, and the reason most people begin the diet in the first place is to facilitate extreme levels of weight loss. The keto diet will enable you to lose weight.

Of course, as with most diets, weight loss in the first few days is mostly water weight. The reason for this is that carbohydrates hold water in the body, and by restricting carbs you don't give the water anything to hold on to in the body. After that, however, the body begins to work on its stored fat to use for fuel and energy. Strictly following a keto diet may assist in controlling the type of diabetes that is caused by weight gain and poor dietary habits. This type of diabetes is a condition marked by high blood pressure, belly fat, and increased blood sugar levels, and has potential health consequences and is known as Type 2 Diabetes. A keto diet can help control these conditions by controlling the levels of sugar and insulin in the bloodstream.

Research has begun that shows that a keto diet might be helpful for patients with Alzheimer's disease by helping to slow the degeneration of brain cells and assisting with better cognitive function in older adults. People with bipolar disorder may experience periods of more stabilized moods by using a keto diet as a mood stabilizer. Early studies suggest that diet may be as important and effective, if not even more so, than medication alone for bipolar disorder. It is also being touted as a treatment for certain cancers. The theory is that, along with chemotherapy and radiation, adhering to a keto diet can provide better nutritional benefits for the patient, giving them more innate energy to fight the effects of the cancer and the conventional treatments. Women with Polycystic Ovary Disease may benefit from the positive benefits of a keto diet since they are at a greater risk of suffering from the effects of obesity and diabetes.

The biggest drawback, perhaps the only real downside to following the keto diet is the brief period of the keto flu, the state where the body reaches ketosis and begins to burn stored fat. The symptoms of ketosis are similar to the symptoms of the flu—nausea and vomiting, headache, tiredness, crankiness, and sometimes vomiting and diarrhea. This is why it is referred to as the keto flu. The symptoms are different for everyone, however. Some people will experience every symptom of keto flu, and some people will sail blithely through this phase with absolutely no problems at all. The best way to combat the effects of the keto flu, which can last for up to a week, is to get plenty of rest, limit physical activity, and stay well hydrated. And always remember that too shall pass.

So how do you know when you have reached the state of ketosis? Is it necessary to just guess, based on how your body feels? The body does give signs that it has entered ketosis. One of these signs is what is known as keto breath. When the body begins to break down fatty acids stored in the liver to use for energy one of the chemicals the body naturally produces is acetone. As a result of the acetone being released from the stored fat, the smell of the breath will begin to change when the body is entering ketosis. This smell has been described as a fruity smell, much like the odor given off by overripe apples. Also, when the body shifts into ketosis, thirst will typically increase. As the body begins to use up excess glycogen stored in the liver, it increases the need for elimination through urination. However, checking for ketosis by measuring how often you urinate is not a valid method of checking for ketosis.

The most accurate way to check to see if your body is in ketosis is by using urine test strips. The test strips are relatively inexpensive, are available at most drug store chains and big box retailers, and using these will allow you to check your ketone levels quickly. If your body is in a state of ketosis, the strip will change its color after being dipped in your urine stream. After using the strip, you will just need to compare it to the color guide on the side of the bottle or box the test strips come in. The entire process takes less than a minute and will give you an accurate reading of what level of ketosis your body has achieved. Just follow the simple instructions that come with whichever brand you chose to purchase.

No diet plan is perfect. The perfect solution would be never to need to follow a weight loss diet ever. But that is not the reality for many of us. Many of us have made poor dietary choices and poor lifestyle choices that have driven us to search for a method to help us turn our bodies and our lives back in the other direction. So if you do feel the need to follow a diet plan, which is most likely why you are here today, the keto diet is your best choice by far. And even though it is often referred to as a diet, it is not so much a diet as a lifestyle change that must be adopted wholeheartedly in order to be completely successful. But do take into consideration that the potential benefits of following the keto diet plan and intermittent fasting far outweigh any inconvenience that may be experienced in the implementation of this diet. Most important of all, don't give up. With careful planning and execution, the keto style of life can benefit anyone.

# Chapter 4: Is Keto and Intermittent Fasting Appropriate for You?

Generally, when people decide to begin a new diet, they begin by first eliminating all the foods in the house that will not be conducive to effective weight loss. Gone are the cookies and cakes, ice cream is banished, and the refrigerator is now filled with an abundance of fresh fruits and vegetables and lean meats. And now the serious dieting phase begins.

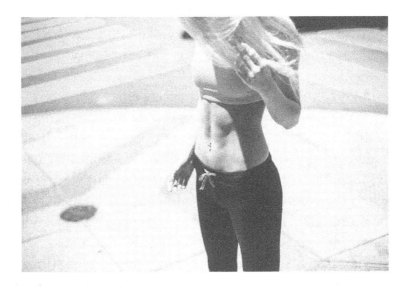

A successful diet plan will motivate you to constantly seek better progress by giving you better results. We were never meant to live without food forever and never to be able to enjoy the food we do eat. But we were also never meant to push an almost non-stop stream of food and drink into our bodies. The keto diet will allow you to keep some of the fatty things that make life so much more enjoyable, and that will give you the fat intake your body craves for flavor, like ranch dressing and sour cream. You will be able to eat bacon, cheese, and steak.

These foods carry enough fat and protein to be particularly useful to the keto dieter and to allow you to stick with your meal plans. Just be prepared to get rid of the breads, the cookies, and the doughnuts. The meal plans of the keto diet will allow you to eat more fats and proteins to help you curb those pesky hunger pains that you will experience from time to time. The most important part of the keto diet is your ability to personalize the meal plans to make them fit into your lifestyle. You have the ability to adjust your keto diet, and your meal plans to be as loose or as rigid as you want and need them to be. You can enable your diet to work at a much faster rate simply by adding intermittent fasting to your regimen. The end result is totally up to you and the personal goals you have set for yourself.

Preparing to embark on a keto diet plan with intermittent fasting is not so different from beginning any other diet plan. Foods that are not allowed on a keto eating plan should be eliminated from your house if possible. It is simply easier for you to follow the eating plan if temptation is not staring you in the face. If the whole house isn't following the same diet plan, it may be more difficult for you to see those cookies and not give in to temptation, but it can be done. Stay strong! And remember that fasting requires no more preparation than selecting the days and times you intend to fast, along with stockpiling a supply of whatever calorie-free beverage you choose to drink to keep yourself well hydrated while fasting.

The keto diet and intermittent fasting will work together well to accelerate weight loss. The processes together also increase many other performance-boosting benefits. Fasting alone is an amazing tool to use to improve your overall health, and adding the keto diet to periods of intermittent fasting will simply rapidly increase the effects. Fasting can be done anytime and everywhere. Keto friendly foods can be found almost anywhere.

So what exactly can combining the keto diet and intermittent fasting do for you? Some of the more well-known health benefits include:

- A rapid reduction in overall body fat
- A decrease in the inflammation that causes pain in the body
- A decrease of the appearance of the effects of aging on the skin
- Faster recovery times after illness or surgery
- Healthier muscle mass and better physical performance
- Improved brain function and cognitive performance

The first most important benefit is the decrease in overall body fat. Combining the positive effects of the keto diet and intermittent fasting will cause the body to begin to use stored fat for energy and fuel. As the stores are used up the body will begin to shrink in size. As the body is no longer stuffed with stores of unhealthy fat, it begins to suffer less from the harmful effects of inflammation. The skin will appear to be healthier and will look softer and suppler. A decrease of body fat by using stored fat for energy leads to an increase in muscle mass and overall better muscular performance. The body is better able to bounce back after surgery or an illness. And better nutritional habits will lead to improved cognitive functioning in the brain.

After beginning the keto diet, you will notice your food cravings will eventually disappear. The regular consumption of fat and protein does not cause unwanted spikes of blood sugar in the blood. As a matter of fact, the keto diet and intermittent fasting used together properly can be instrumental in curing Type 2 Diabetes in some people. This type of diabetes is a direct result of obesity and poor dietary choices. Put the keto diet together with intermittent fasting and you have a powerful tool to help keep your blood sugar levels steady at all times, thus eliminating the rises and falls that leads to those intense food cravings that cause you to make poor choices.

The keto diet suppresses hunger, even during times of intermittent fasting. Following the keto diet forces the body to tap into hidden stores of glycogen stored in the liver to use as fuel for the other cells in the body. When this happens, the body produces ketones to break down the pockets of stored fat. Ketone production suppresses ghrelin, which is the body's main hunger hormone and responsible for those annoying hunger pains. But while you are on the keto diet, your hunger is naturally suppressed even when food is not being consumed. Since hunger pains are suppressed or even eliminated, you can go longer periods without consuming food, thus prompting the body into an even greater capacity for weight loss.

Using the keto diet together with periods of intermittent fasting will automatically increase fat loss even if calories are not restricted. The weight will come off quite quickly with minimal effort. While on the keto diet you can use the benefits of intermittent fasting to counteract binge eating.

Intermittent fasting allows you to set up your fasting schedule to suit your particular needs and lifestyle. You have the freedom to set up your fasting schedule to fast on alternate days, or for a set time daily. The choice is totally yours to decide. Following the keto diet helps to regulate your blood sugar, and that one small step alone will help to prevent higher blood pressure and heart problems. Research also suggests that a side benefit of the keto diet is sharper mental abilities. That is definitely something to think about.

Before starting the keto diet and intermittent fasting, there are certain things to take into consideration. Not everyone is well suited to either or both of these forms of weight loss. If your body isn't ready for such a diet, you can actually do more harm than good by starting these plans.

The first most obvious sign that you are not ready for keto and intermittent fasting is recent or impending motherhood. The keto diet and intermittent fasting are not recommended for expectant mothers. During pregnancy, your body naturally requires more carbohydrates for energy and fuel than is readily available when following the keto diet. You are feeding a baby, a living human being, inside your body. Every food and drink item that you consume during this time will be used by the body to feed the baby first. Your nutrition needs to be well round and just plentiful enough to provide nutrients for both baby and mother. There will be time enough after the baby is born to get started on a weight loss and fasting routine, but if you are currently pregnant, please be patient, feed your baby, and keep this in mind for the future. If you are a new mother who is nursing, this also may not be the plan for you. The restrictive calorie intact and fasting may not provide enough calories for you to continue making nutritious milk for your new baby. Again, take care of the baby and keep this plan in mind for your future post-baby body.

People with Type 1 Diabetes are definitely not good candidates for either a keto diet or intermittent fasting. Type 1 Diabetes, formerly called Juvenile Diabetes, is an actual medical condition that must be carefully controlled with diet and medication. Those with Type 2 Diabetes, generally thought of as adult-onset diabetes, could benefit greatly from a keto diet and fasting to lose weight because obesity is one of the major causes of Type 2 Diabetes.

Those with kidney or liver disease may not be good candidates for undertaking the keto diet and intermittent fasting. Since the body will be producing chemicals in the liver that will facilitate the removal of wastes through the kidneys, both of these organs may be stressed by the keto diet and intermittent fasting.

Anyone who is currently suffering from any type of eating disorder, such as anorexia or bulimia, should think carefully before beginning a keto diet or intermittent fasting, as these may not be appropriate for people with those conditions. Any eating disorder that takes your mental image of yourself and your body and transfers it to a physical phenomenon will not be cured by the keto diet or by intermittent fasting. It will first be necessary to correct the thoughts and ideas that are leading to your negative body image before attempting a diet that will change your existing body image.

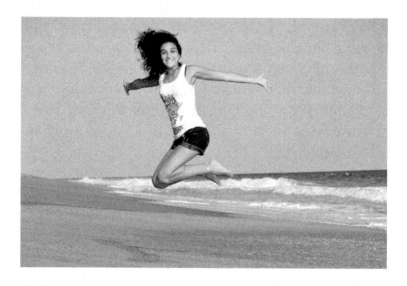

Unfortunately, people with underlying major medical conditions, such as muscular dystrophy, are probably not good candidates for the keto diet plan and intermittent fasting. Severe conditions such as these may require a diet plan and nutritional intake that cannot be met by the more restrictive keto diet, and fasting may be contraindicated for those whose nutritional needs are greater because of a disease or condition they, unfortunately, suffer from.

Children who are under the age of eighteen are definitely not good candidates for the keto diet and intermittent fasting. Growing children have specific dietary needs to help them to grow and develop properly. Children who suffer from obesity need to be under the care of a personal physician to help them lose excess weight while still maintaining the nutritional requirements they have. Older teens may be able to safely do the diet and fasting with close supervision since they have basically grown to their full personal potential, but it definitely is not recommended for small children. Little ones have needs that may not be met by the keto diet, and going without food for an extended period of time would not be beneficial to their health and well-being.

Have you recently undergone major surgery? You may not be a good candidate for beginning the keto diet or intermittent fasting, at least in the early days just after your surgery. The first days after surgery usually require extremely good nutrition to assist the body in rebuilding cells needed for you to make a complete recovery. Take the time you need to get back to one hundred percent function before attempting a keto diet or intermittent fasting.

Those who take medication for a chronic condition should also proceed with caution. Certain foods sometimes react with certain medication with an adverse reaction. Your pharmacist can advise you if there are any dietary restrictions you must follow with the medication you are currently taking.

This list may seem daunting, but it really isn't. Most people will be able to begin using the keto diet plan and intermittent fasting to aid in their personal weight loss goals. As with any diet program, it is best to know any possible limitations before beginning the program and finding out that it will not work for you. If you are in reasonably good health, with no serious underlying medical conditions and no unrealistic body image issues, then you will definitely benefit greatly from using the keto diet and intermittent fasting to help you reach and maintain your personal weight loss goals.

# Chapter 5: Things You Need to Know to Make the Keto Diet Work for You

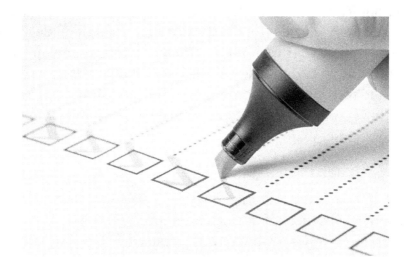

Beginning your journey to better health by using the keto diet plan is definitely not quite the same as beginning any other basic weight loss program where you take in fewer calories to help facilitate weight loss. You do not just wake up one day and decide to suddenly begin eating according to the keto way. There are many different facets to the keto diet that you must know before beginning to help you make the best possible choices and achieve the best possible outcome.

Let's begin by talking about ketosis. Ketosis is the process that occurs when the body begins to produce ketones in the liver. This process is a by-product of the body tearing into stored fat in search of energy and fuel for the body and the mind. The state of ketosis is similar to the flu in the symptoms it produces—headache, nausea and vomiting, lethargy, and irritability.

These symptoms can, unfortunately, plague you for up to a

week, but when they are gone, and your body has adjusted to the lowered carbohydrate consumption level, then good things start to happen in terms of increased energy and mental function. Your body will remain in the state of ketosis unless you suddenly decide to drastically increase, then decrease, them increase, your carb intake. If you do this, then your body will need to go through ketosis again to enable you to get back to a state where you are continuously burning stored fat. That is why this is often referred to as a style of life change and not a temporary diet plan.

The ketones that are produced during the process of ketosis are small bits of fuel that the body will use for energy in the temporary absence of a regular supply of food. The body produces ketones when you restrict the amount of carbohydrates you eat. Carbohydrates are the number one source of sugar supplies in the blood. Excess protein will also be converted to blood sugar if more protein is consumed that the body needs to use at that moment, so it will be necessary to constantly keep your protein intake within the recommended guidelines for the keto eating plan. These ketones that the body produces are used by all the cells in your body for fuel and energy. Even the brain will use ketones to fuel its processes.

The body has limited supplies of readily available ketones to use for energy and fuel. When these stores have been exhausted the body will turn to its stores of fat for fuel and energy. Insulin is the hormone that your body naturally produces in response to food consumption that helps the body store more food as fat. When you eat carbohydrates, the body automatically uses insulin to convert the bulk of these carbs into sugar. When you do not eat carbs the body automatically produces less insulin, for it knows that an excessive flow of insulin is not needed. If the body is not producing insulin to store food into fat, it prompts the body to turn to fat stores for fuel and energy. This is how we begin to lose weight on the keto diet.

Our bodies have evolved to become very smart, very efficient machines if we allow them to do things the way they were meant to do them. Even a relatively lean person has enough stored fat to fuel the body for a long period of time before starvation begins. The body's process of using ketosis to supply fuel and energy also guarantees that the brain will have enough fuel to sustain its life and allow it to function normally.

The state of ketosis will occur at the beginning of using any version of the keto diet if the diet is followed properly and little to no cheating occurs. Several versions of the keto diet plan exist and are in use today. There are the high-protein ketogenic diet plan and the standard ketogenic diet plan. These two variations are the ones most often used by individuals seeking weight loss and improved health. The other two types, the targeted ketogenic diet plan, and the cyclical ketogenic diet plan are both highly specialized diet plans usually reserved for those with higher nutritional needs, such as athletes or bodybuilders in training.

Similar to the standard keto diet, the high-protein ketogenic diet has a higher level of protein intake. This form of the diet allows the user to consume a diet that is five percent carbs, thirty-five percent proteins, and sixty percent fat. This option might be the best one for people who have a naturally higher need for more dietary protein, such as larger men, athletes, and anyone who regularly performs hard physical labor. Also, some people just naturally feel better when they consume larger amounts of protein. The ratio can be used as a guideline and experimented with to best meet your particular dietary needs.

If you are following the high-protein keto diet plan, you will intake slightly more protein than is allowed on the standard keto diet. This plan is best for bodybuilders needing increased muscle mass, and aging people who may be losing muscle mass. On this keto diet plan, you will consume a bit more protein than on the standard keto diet plan. On this plan you will get thirty percent of your food calories from proteins, sixty-five percent will come from the consumption of fats, and five percent will come from eating carbohydrates.

You will want to get the bulk of your protein from fish, meat, and poultry. People who have kidney problems are probably not good candidates for this keto eating plan. Taking in too much protein might cause a buildup of waste products in the kidneys. And if your intended benefit is something therapeutic, then the high-protein plan may not be the right one for you. If you are following a keto diet to treat or hopefully eliminate seizures, then the higher protein levels may not allow you to build up a high enough level of ketones in your body to be helpful to you. A slightly higher level of protein in the diet will not be enough to kick your body out of a state of ketosis, so this plan should give the average person the same effects and results as the standard keto diet.

The targeted keto diet plan is one of the more flexible forms of keto dieting. You are able to add more carbs into the diet to coincide with times when you are working out. It is the perfect plan for anyone who finds the standard keto diet too restrictive or lacking in a carbohydrate count high enough to meet their nutritional needs. It is often used by athletes and bodybuilders. It is the perfect method for adding more carbs into the diet after being in a period of strict ketosis. It is of the utmost importance that you are in a state of strict ketosis before transitioning to the targeted keto diet, for a period of at least sixty days. This amount of time will give the body enough time to become what is known as 'fat adapted' where your body will know how to use incoming glucose quickly and efficiently. This is important because high levels of carbohydrates will turn to sugar in the body and are generally stored as fat.

On the targeted keto plan, you will follow the diet restrictions completely until about one hour before indulging in intensive physical activity—before you exercise. At that time, you will quickly consume about twenty-five grams of carbs. This will allow your body to have sufficient carbs to use as fuel and energy during your workout, while still allowing the body to quickly return to ketosis after you have finished your workout. The key is to consume carbs that are easily digestible in a very short time, such as a slice of white bread or a small bowl of white rice. This plan is best for those who regularly engage in high energy physical activity. This would apply to bodybuilders, marathon swimmers, and cross-country runners.

This plan is not meant for those who go to the gym to engage in their regularly scheduled moderate workout.

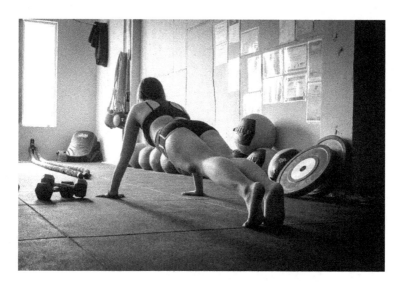

On the cyclical ketogenic diet plan, the user is allowed to choose to rotate days of high carb intake and days of low carb intake in a cycle that best suits their particular style of life. Are you currently training for a marathon on your days off from work? Then you might benefit from a higher carb intake on those days only. Are you working in a warehouse three days a week for fifteen hours each day? Then you might want to increase your carb intake on the days when you work and lower it on your days off. The cyclical diet plan might take a bit more planning than the standard keto diet plan, but it is workable, especially if it better suits your particular dietary needs. This plan is best for anyone who really finds it difficult sticking to a very low carb keto diet. This plan will allow you to take a temporary break and enjoy a few extra carbohydrates every now and then. The biggest problem with this plan is that it might cause you to go on a huge carb binge and ruin all the wonderful progress you have already made.

It is best to avoid trying to use this plan until your body has fully adapted to the keto way of life and have been in a state of ketosis for at least a period of sixty days. It is of the utmost importance that you plan to give your body enough time to adjust to this new way of eating and to give your body a chance to get back to working at maximum efficiency. And, since carbs hold water in the body, this plan may lead to internal fluid fluctuations and may not be advisable for people with underlying heart conditions.

The plan most often used by those who follow keto is called the standard ketogenic diet plan. On this plan, you will consume a high amount of fats, a moderate amount of proteins, and a low amount of carbohydrates. The ratio is generally five percent carbohydrates, seventy-five percent fats, and twenty percent protein. This is calculated by determining the overall calorie count of the foods involved in the meal, then dividing those calories into the proper category.

No discussion of keto dieting and intermittent fasting would be complete without a discussion on autophagy. Although this term is not usually discussed, it is a very important component of the ketogenic diet. During autophagy, the cells in the body start using the little damaged and defective bits floating around inside themselves to rebuild healthy cells from formerly damaged cells. The cells are basically using their own bits of trash as fuel to improve their own inner workings. Autophagy is not limited to periods of intermittent fasting. It is a process that occurs daily with the cells in the body but at a much slower rate. And the process is generally suppressed in the bodies of obese people since the cells are not allowed to go through the normal cellular processes. This process can be accelerated by the use of intermittent fasting. The normal process of autophagy reaches its maximum peak of effectiveness around twelve to sixteen hours into the fasting period. The body maintains this peak for about two days. So to achieve the maximum benefits from autophagy you should plan to wait no more than forty-eight hours before beginning another intermittent fasting period.

The process of autophagy can be accelerated by using protein cycling. Consuming fats and proteins instead of carbs will spark the beginning of autophagy. Protein cycling, the practice of consuming more proteins than normal on certain days and less on other days, will cause the process of autophagy to happen even faster. In the case of autophagy, the intermittent fast is actually the preferred method for jump-starting the process. Autophagy will occur at the beginning of a longer, sustained fast, but this process requires a regular influx of vitamins and nutrients to allow the body to repeat the cycle at maximum effectiveness. The profound lack of food in a longer fast does not allow for replenishment of nutrition to the cells. Thus autophagy will not work as well as it normally would without fasting and the process may even be slower than normal.

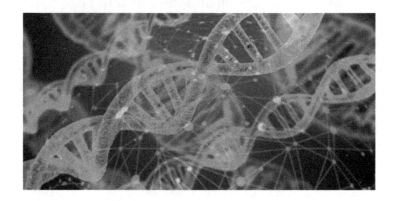

Since the main object of using the keto diet and practicing intermittent fasting is usually to lose weight, how much weight can you expect to lose during this lifestyle change? Well, that depends. Under normal circumstances, anyone who takes in less food, such as while fasting, will automatically lose weight. Every pound of body weight depends on the physical makeup of the human who is taking in the calories. A pound of fat is fueled by roughly 3500 calories. So if you cut about one thousand calories out of your daily diet, you could lose one to two pounds every week.

Since no one becomes obese overnight, a one to two pound reduction every week is respectable progress. You will slowly teach your body to adjust to a lower calorie intake and be happy with potentially less food. However, many people are frustrated by the slow progress and give up after a few weeks, not understanding that they should think of this as a change of lifestyle and not a temporary diet because no one is able to diet forever. Granted, at the rate of one to two pounds per week it could take you almost seven months to lose fifty pounds. But, remember, no one became overweight overnight.

The major benefit of the keto lifestyle is that it will jump start your weight loss as soon as your body enters the state of ketosis and you force your body to use existing fat stores as fuel. During the first week or two, you might lose anywhere from two to ten or twenty pounds. Remember this will be mostly water weight loss, for a very specific reason. The body uses water to hold carbs in the cells. When the carbohydrate intake is lowered, the body turns to glycogen stored in the cells to burn for energy. When these glycogen stores have been depleted the body has no more need to store excess water and will flush it out of the body through the kidneys. Good hydration is essential during this time. Don't worry; the body won't store the extra liquid. It will use what it needs and flush out the rest.

After the initial water-flushing period, weight loss may slow as the body begins to almost completely use stored fat for energy. Now you can expect to lose anywhere from one to five pounds weekly. This may not sound like much, especially when compared to the one to two pound loss on a regular diet. So why is keto dieting and intermittent fasting so much better for you?

Two pounds lost on a regular diet is two pounds lost. It might be fat, and it might be muscle. It might only be water weight. After you reach the state of ketosis, two pounds lost on a keto diet is two pounds of fat, as the body begins to use it stores. The difference is that one pound of fat is physically larger than one pound of muscle. If your body is definitely losing fat stores, then your overall body measurements will shrink.

So while the scale might not record an actual loss of pounds that is compatible with what you thought it should be, your waistline will definitely be getting smaller, and you will find your clothes will begin to fit much better.

It is also worthy to note that different people will lose weight at different rates. This is something most people do not take into consideration when their diet plan does not work as well as they think it should. Men will usually naturally lose weight faster than women because of the hormone testosterone, which gives men the naturally leaner, more muscular body. Women generally have an abundance of estrogen, a hormone that promotes weight retention and gain. Women, who were meant to carry babies within their bodies, are genetically predisposed to hold onto weight longer so that we can deliver healthy babies during times when food is scarce or unavailable. Younger people will naturally lose weight faster than older people, simply because their metabolism runs at a faster rate. Morbidly obese people will lose weight faster than someone who weighs less at the beginning of the diet because they naturally have more fat stores and more to lose. It is very important to understand the different factors that come together to make your personal self so that you can use this knowledge to maximize your weight loss goals.

Careful planning must be maintained if the keto diet is to be successful for you.

In the beginning adherence to a keto diet may seem overwhelming at first, but it is not an impossible task. Your main focus will be finding ways to reduce your carbohydrate intake while increasing the overall fat and protein content of your meals and snacks. Carbohydrate consumption must be continuously restricted if you are to ever reach a state of ketosis. Most people will need to consume less than twenty grams of carbs each day to successfully reach ketosis. Generally speaking, the lower you set and keep your total net carb intake daily, the faster you will begin burning those pesky leftover fat stores to start revealing the new and improved you. Sticking to keto friendly foods and meal plans designed to avoid over-consumption of carbs is the best way to be successful on a keto diet.

So exactly what would a sample keto menu look like? I have included a few here to give you an idea of what this eating plan looks like in reality.

- Breakfast—scrambled eggs and bacon
  Lunch—Ham and cheese roll ups, cottage cheese, olives
  Dinner—Chicken thighs with cabbage and cheese

- Breakfast—Keto blueberry muffins with scrambled eggs
  Lunch—Philly cheesesteak roll up
  Dinner—Bowl of egg roll

- Breakfast—Eggs in pepper rings
  Lunch—shrimp salad
  Dinner—Grilled kebobs

- Breakfast—Keto pancakes
  Lunch—Easy meatballs
  Dinner—Chicken breast supreme

- Breakfast—Smooth fruit smoothie
  Lunch—Tuna wraps
  Dinner—Fish sticks

These are just a few suggestions. The recipes for these menu items and many more can be located at the end of this book in the recipe section I have provided to help you get started. The possible combinations of menu items are endless. In the beginning, until you are used to what twenty grams of carbs look like or how to determine a serving of meat or chicken, it is best to weigh and measure your food portions and to follow the recipes strictly. This may take longer in the beginning, but you will soon learn what portions should look like and how to calculate your carbohydrate count for the day. When you have become better at eyeballing portions and knowing what is and is not allowed, you will be able to experiment with your meal choices, adding and removing food items to suit your particular dietary needs and preferences. Just remember no meal suggestion is set in stone. If you are planning dinner and the meal plan you have chosen calls for a side of asparagus and you absolutely despise asparagus, then you are probably not going to eat half of your meal. In those instances, it is perfectly acceptable to combine two recipes and prepare the side salad or vegetable medley bowl that you see on the next recipe. No recipe will be effective if you refuse to eat the food suggested.

It is important to pay strict attention to your meal plans and food choices in the beginning especially. You must make absolutely certain that your protein/fat/carb ratio is kept exactly to the standards for every day. You will need to find a way to track your meals. Whether you download a tracking app, write things down in a notebook, or build an elaborate spreadsheet, you will need to find the method that works for you and stick to it until you are very experienced with keto. And do not think the keto diet is a license to gorge yourself on cheeses and meats. If you do a computer search for keto recipes, this is likely what you will find. But it is just as important to work in your allowed vegetables on a daily basis. They will be what keep certain systems in the body moving in the way they should. And you might find that cooking many meals at one time, or cooking all your meat for the week at one time, will make sticking to the diet much easier. Do not give up if it does not work perfectly at first. You will get this right.

The important thing to remember is that this is a lifestyle change. You must take all available information and use your knowledge to your advantage. Instead of feeling overwhelmed by the great amount of information, take the time to read everything possible so that you know exactly what will be expected of you to be successful, and exactly the results you can expect to see. Only by being fully informed can you hope to be successful in this new lifestyle.

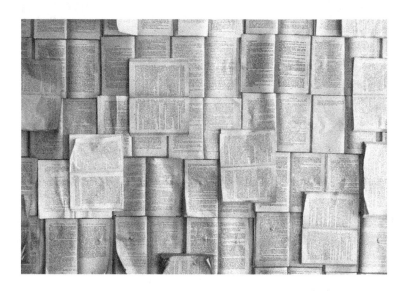

# Chapter 6: Combining the Keto Diet and Intermittent Fasting for Maximum Weight Loss

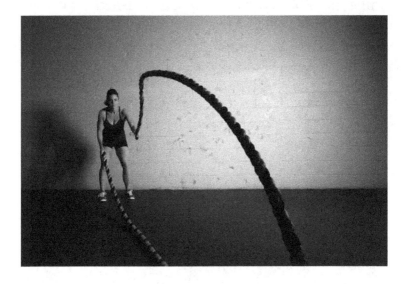

So if keto is a way of eating and intermittent fasting is a way of not eating, can the two be combined in a plan to maximize weight loss? Definitely! By using the strategies of the keto eating lifestyle along with intermittent fasting, you can be successful on this plan.

It is so amazing how much good that intermittent fasting can do for the human body. There are many benefits associated with intermittent fasting. When you eat all your meals in a time-specific window or only on certain days you automatically take in less food. Therefore you take in fewer calories, which will automatically lead to weight loss.

And recent studies suggest that those people fast while consuming a healthy diet lose weight at least twice as fast as those who fast and continue to eat poorly.

The human body is only comfortable eating so much food at any one time. We, as humans, with eyes bigger than our stomachs, continuously push that envelope and regularly stuff more and even more food into our poor little tummies. Since the body only needs a certain number of calories to perform its daily duties, any food that is not eliminated as waste is stored as fat. So we might as well rub that extra piece of cake right on our hip because that is where it will eventually end up. So we routinely build up these marvelous fat stores that cause us to feel sluggish and inefficient in our movements and routines. And the smaller window of opportunity for eating that fasting naturally gives us eliminates unnecessary snacking, especially during those late hours just before bed.

By following the high-fat low-carb keto diet, the body experiences lower levels of hunger and faster, greater feelings of fullness. It is so much easier and more pleasant to follow an intermittent fasting schedule when you do not feel as though you are starving to death.

In the beginning, intermittent fasting may not make you feel very comfortable. You are probably dying from starvation. You feel you must rush into the kitchen and eat everything in sight. Remember to allow yourself an adequate period of time to adjust to fasting. Your body will eventually adjust, and you will not starve in the meantime. You will happily discover that as time goes on and you become more used to the keto diet and the periods of fasting that you will naturally not be as hungry as you were before.

Intermittent fasting is not a part of ketogenic dieting, but it is a natural component to the diet. It is a compatible and definitely recommended way to boost your personal weight loss goals.

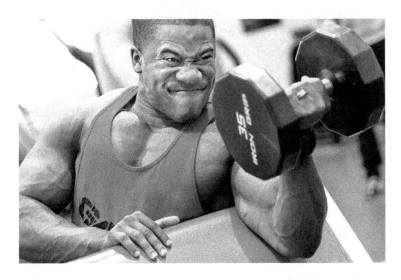

Fasting for just twenty-four hours has a remarkable effect on the muscular system by increasing the levels of human growth hormone in the body. This hormone is responsible for enabling us to grow and maintain strong muscles. So there is no need to worry that weight loss will lead automatically to a loss of muscle tissue and overall body weakness. Higher levels of human growth hormones also lead to thicker bone density and lower overall body fat levels.

Let's face it—aging happens to the best of us. Skin begins to lose its elasticity, causing wrinkles and sags in places we least expect. Human growth hormone helps the human body to keep more collagen in the skin, thus keeping skin thicker and more resistant to those pesky wrinkles.

Intermittent fasting also increases the rate at which stem cells are produced in the body. Since the human body can use stem cells for any purpose, you could think of them as biological playdough. The human body will use stem cells to replace old cells and damaged cells. Replacing these old or damaged cells will keep the body younger on a cellular level and better able to cope with normal wear and tear the body suffers on a daily basis. Stem cells can be used to replace dying cells in the skin, keeping that youthful appearance longer. Stem cells can be used by our joints to replace dying connective tissue, making our joints stronger longer and hopefully putting off those dreaded joint replacement surgeries.

Intermittent fasting is an excellent therapy for the brain. When you fast, your body increases production of proteins in the brain that help the brain increase its ability to learn and remember. It can also help your brain keep current thought pathways strong and to build new ones in the event of injury, which is especially important as we age and become more susceptible to age-related issues like strokes.

Using intermittent fasting properly provides a system-wide tune up for the entire body. And it makes sense that the body performs better during fasting. When you think of it from the viewpoint of evolution, the times when the food supply is scarce are the exact times when the body and mind need to work in a more sharply focused manner to enable us to find food quickly.

But why do you need to follow a keto diet while doing intermittent fasting? Won't any diet work the same way? Is it really necessary to change your entire way of eating to make this fasting thing work properly? The answer is yes. The problem with fasting while eating a regular, higher carbohydrate diet is that carbs stay in the body longer and generally turn into sugars and then into fat. This can lead to an imbalance in the level of sugar in the blood and cause problems associated with high or low blood sugar. By combining intermittent fasting with a keto diet, you allow the body to consume good, healthy foods that will provide energy and fuel for the body throughout the period of the fast until food will be consumed again.

By using the keto diet, you stop eating excess amounts of carbs and replace those food items with fat and protein. When your body begins to adjust to eating fewer carbohydrates, it will become much more efficient at burning excess fat stores to use as fuel. The body will spend all its time in a delicious fat burning state, constantly pumping energy throughout the body.

Using the keto diet is also a great way to suppress hunger. When eating the keto way, the liver begins to break down stored fat to use as magical little bursts of energy for the body to consume. The ketones that are produced by the liver also work to suppress the feelings of hunger that drive us to overeat. While on the keto diet the body's hunger hormones are effectively suppressed, even when food is not being actively consumed. You can easily sail through longer periods of not eating without feeling deprived or starved.

Always make sure you are consuming healthy high-fat food. Junk food has no place in the keto lifestyle. You will be eating less often. You will be eating less food as a total amount. For these reasons, it is vital that your food intake be as nutritious as possible. Do not overlook your fiber intake. Do not cut back on your good fat intake. And do not forget your veggies. A good way to avoid feeling totally lost is to start with either the keto dieting or intermittent fasting first, then to add the other one in. If you feel strong enough to do both and want to make a clean break with your old lifestyle, then, by all means, begin both at the same time. If you have never fasted before, or if it has been awhile, you might want to start with a shorted fast, such as your sleeping hours plus four more hours. People who sleep the recommended number of hours per night say seven to eight hours of sleep, will be able to do the bulk of their fasting while sleeping. When you grow more comfortable with fasting, then feel free to add on even more hours.

It is necessary to reiterate that no one diet plan will fit every individual. As each person is a varied and unique human being, so too does each person require a diet plan that suits them. As with dieting, fasting also needs to be tailored to the individual and what is best for them. By personalizing your diet plan with those keto recipes and meals you find most appealing, and by arranging your fasting schedule to fit into your personal life, you will more readily set yourself up for success.

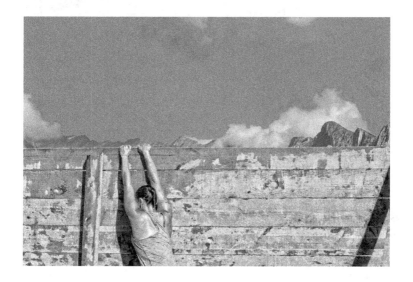

# Chapter 7: Lifestyle Changes to Maximize Dietary Changes

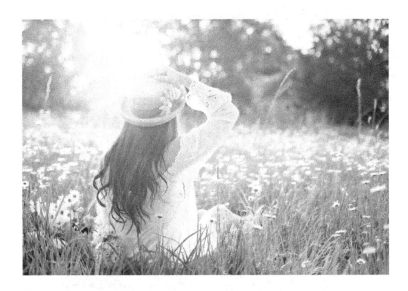

So what does one need to do to successfully jump start this new lifestyle of the keto diet and intermittent fasting? Some changes definitely need to be made in order to maximize weight loss and your chances of success. You can't expect to be successful at this by walking in half prepared. Starting the keto diet is not like starting any other diet plan. The keto diet will require meticulous planning and preparation. But you can do this!

The first change happens even before starting the new diet. Begin by keeping a food diary for two weeks. Write down everything you eat and drink, and when you eat or drink it. This is not a book of shame or a listing of all the things you do to yourself that are bad.

You will never need to show this book to anyone else if you do not want to. This will be for your eyes only. This food diary is merely a tool to let you see exactly when you eat, how often and how much. By keeping a list, you will see exactly what you are putting into your body and when.

This will also assist you when setting up your intermittent fasting schedule. It is easier to plan your times of fasting if you have a better understanding of when you do and do not eat.

After keeping your two-week food diary, spend some time looking through it. Grab a highlighter and highlight all the times food was consumed that was not a protein or a vegetable. Now, look at what you've highlighted. Keep in mind that cookies, cakes, pies, ice cream, cold cereals, and most fruits will not be included in your new diet plan. They are all way too high in carbohydrates and will cause you to fail in your weight loss efforts.

The next step is to go through your kitchen and purge it of all the foods you will no longer be eating. Get rid of the sugary treats, the boxes of breakfast cereal, the snack cakes in the cabinet, the ice cream treats in the freezer and all that fruit that is not a part of the keto diet. Don't throw it away, but do donate anything you can to a food bank or a family member. If you've just done the weekly shopping, perhaps it would be better to wait until you've consumed some of these stores of food. A few days delay in beginning your new way of life won't necessarily hurt you. Just don't buy any more of these foods. And do not use a temporary delay as an excuse to put of beginning forever. This delay is just temporary.

Maintaining a keto diet will require more dietary changes than merely getting rid of certain foods and beverages, so they no longer tempt you. You must have a good understanding of how various foods fit into the keto diet. One of the biggest questions people have is whether or not a particular food is keto friendly and will it fit into my keto meal plan. Well, let's look at a few examples.

Consider the lowly apple, a beautiful, tasty gift from nature. An average medium-sized apple has twenty-five grams of carbs and four grams of fiber. When counting carbs, you need to remover the number of grams of fiber from the overall carbohydrate count. In this case, twenty-five minus four equals twenty-one. So the apple has twenty-one grams of net carbs. Net carbs are the carbs that your body will turn into fat stores given half a chance. Generally speaking, net carbs should account for no more than five percent of your daily overall calorie intake, which translates to about twenty-five grams of carbohydrates. Since the apple only has twenty-one grams of net carbs, it fits right into our equation. Or does it?

Now, take into consideration the foods you will eat during the remainder of the day. You only have four grams of net carbs left for the entire remainder of all the meals for this day. This means that for the rest of the day if you eat that apple, all your calories will need to come from meat, fish, hard cheese, and eggs—all foods that don't have carbs. This might be fine to do occasionally; sometimes you just really want to have that buttery biscuit. Just keep in mind that the net carb total of twenty-five must last you for an entire day of eating. Because while it is okay once in a while, consuming all your net carbs in one food item on a regular basis is a really bad idea. Doing so will force you to make poor nutritional choices for the remainder of the day and may cause you to miss vital nutrients and vitamins that you would otherwise get from a varied diet.

Is it necessary to count calories on the keto diet? Well, yes and no. If you are comfortable keeping to a strict meal plan and only eating the amounts specified by the daily plan, then you probably will not need to count calories. But when on the keto diet, especially in the beginning, it may be difficult to stick to a portion-controlled plan or even to fully understand what that plan should look like. If one piece of chicken is good for me wouldn't two be better? It's a protein, right? Well yes, the chicken is a carb free protein, but it also has calories. It will do you no good to eat only healthy foods if you continue to eat too much food. Calories count too. So it's not a bad idea, especially in the beginning, to occasionally look at the number of calories you consume in a day and make sure it isn't so high it will sabotage all your good effort. Besides, consuming fat and protein will make you feel less hungry. The body needs to work harder to digest fats and proteins, so you will feel fuller longer by eliminating most carbs from your diet.

It may be particularly difficult to stay on the keto diet when you are away from home. It does require more planning, but it isn't impossible. Any restaurant that features breakfast items is a great place for a keto dieter to eat. Eggs and bacon are good sources of protein, and bacon provides necessary fat. Just tell the waitress to hold the toast, and don't order that tiny glass of orange juice, no matter how good it might taste. Black coffee or tea will be your beverage of choice. For lunch and dinner, the choices are even more abundant. A chef's salad will provide you with good carbs in the form of lettuce, and the meat, egg, and cheese are great sources of protein. Just ask for dressing on the side, preferably ranch. Oil and vinegar is also a good choice for dressing your salad. Order your meat item ala carte. A portion of fish, chicken, or beef will provide protein without blowing your carbohydrate count for the day. Even a cheeseburger without the bun is a decent choice. A piece of meat with a small side salad is a perfectly acceptable keto meal. For snacks on the go, string cheese or hard-boiled eggs are always a good choice.

Fitting intermittent fasting into your life is actually easier than maintaining your keto diet. After all, with fasting, you merely need to decide when you will and will not eat. Make sure it fits into your particular schedule, or you will not be setting yourself up for success. It's best to plan to bulk of your fasting for when you will naturally be asleep. So if you eat your dinner meal at six in the evening, begin fasting at seven and continue it through the overnight hours. A sixteen hour fast will take you through to eleven the next morning. Most people don't jump out of bed and head right for the kitchen to grab something to eat. If you start your day at five, six, or seven there are very few hours left until the first meal of the day. Grab some coffee or tea, without cream or sugar. This should help keep you satisfied until lunchtime. It won't be as easy in the very beginning, but your body will adjust. And many people do regularly skip eating breakfast without any adverse effects on their body or their day.

It is not impossible to work the keto diet and intermittent fasting into your life. The biggest problem you will face is eating. More specifically, eating out. It is possible to eat restaurant foods while on the keto diet, but it is more difficult and should be kept to a minimum in the beginning. We are social creatures and love to meet our friends for coffee or drinks, but going forward alcoholic beverages are definitely not allowed, and your coffee must be taken black, no sugar. No more lattes! When you embark on this lifestyle change, you will be faced with many new challenges. But conquering them is the first step toward weight loss success and the new you.

# Chapter 8: Good Foods and Bad Foods

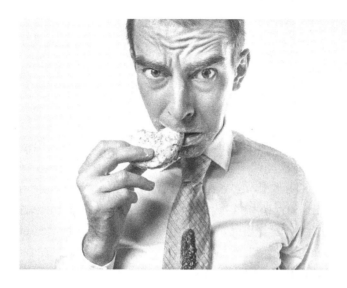

To maintain a healthy relationship with food we are encouraged to never think of food as good or bad. Food is nourishment for the body. Food is necessary for maintaining life as we know it. There really are no bad foods if all foods are consumed in moderation.

However, we are discussing beginning the keto diet, which means that at some point you have over-indulged in eating certain if not all, foods and you now find it necessary to restrict food intake in such a way that will allow you to lose weight and feel healthy again.

The keto diet requires intaking certain foods and avoiding certain foods in order to facilitate ketosis and stay on track with the requirements of the diet. The most important thing to remember is that the keto diet is a low carbohydrate plan. That means that no more than twenty-five to thirty-five grams of carbohydrates will be consumed on a daily basis. Sticking to this requirement is important for several reasons. By restricting carbs, you force the liver to produce ketones that, in turn, attack the body's fat stores looking for energy. This will send your body into ketosis, which is when your body begins to maximize its fat burning abilities. It is important to keep your carb count down every day. If you allow your carb count to creep back up, then your body will come out of ketosis and will no longer burn fat for fuel.

So how do you figure your net carbs? This is where reading food labels helps. A net carb is the grams of carbohydrate count minus the grams of fiber count. For example, consider the apple. A medium apple has twenty-five grams of carbohydrates and four grams of fiber. Twenty-five minus four equals twenty-one. So an apple has twenty-one grams of net carbs. Not bad in reality, but not good on the low carb keto diet.

So let's look at the food we would consider 'good' for the keto diet, those foods that are allowed, even welcomed, on the keto diet.

Beginning at the produce counter, fill your cart with all the lettuces—iceberg, romaine, leaf, watercress, field greens.

Greens are good for you, so look for turnip greens, collard greens, kale, mustard greens, and spinach. Good individual vegetables include tomatoes, radishes, mushrooms, eggplant, asparagus, avocados, celery, cucumbers, green beans, and cabbage. Remember, for vegetables you want to look for ones that grow above the ground as they tend to be lower in carbohydrates.

As far as fruits go, the only ones that really fit well into the keto diet are the berries—strawberries, raspberries, blackberries, and blueberries. All other fruits tend to be too high in fruit sugar which means they are high in carbs.

Going around to the meat counter, you will find the keto dieter's paradise. Here there are many no-carb and very-low-carb choices. Look for chicken, turkey, beef, and pork, all forms. Here is where you will find bacon, a food that provides both protein and fat. Hot dogs and sausage are also good choices, just read the label and steer clear of added sugars. Fatty fish, whitefish, shrimp, lobster, oysters, and crab will round out your seafood selections. There is a treasure trove at the deli counter to include sliced ham and chicken, roast beef, pepperoni, and salami. You will also find prepared tuna salad, egg salad, and chicken salad. Again, read the labels to look for and avoid added sugar.

In the dairy case, you will find real butter and heavy cream. Eggs are wonderful. Good soft cheeses include provolone, Swiss, cream cheese, brie, and Colby. Hard cheeses found here include parmesan, Havarti, pepper jack, and cheddar. You will also find full-fat sour cream, ricotta cheese, cottage cheese, and yogurt.

In the center area of the store don't forget to look for olive oil, canned chicken and tuna, olives, pickles, mustard, mayonnaise, broth, pork rinds, club soda, and tea and coffee.

So what do we want to avoid on the keto diet? We want to avoid those foods that are high carbohydrate foods that will ruin our ketosis and totally eliminate any progress we might be making. Those foods are what brought us here in the first place.

Sugar is the first big no-no. This means no soft drinks, vitamin waters, sports drinks, and fruit juices. Avoid the aisle in the center of the store that holds all the cookies, cake mixes, snack cakes, frosting, canned fruit, donuts, and candies. There is nothing on this aisle for you. Also, avoid the cereal aisle. Cold cereals, breakfast bars, and any manner of flavored toaster treat are now off limits.

There will be no bread in any form, no rolls, no buns, and no sandwich bread. You will not consume rice, pasta, or potatoes. Say goodbye to potato chips. Beans and root vegetables (other than green beans) are high in carbohydrates. Beer is nothing more than liquid bread. And never buy margarine.

The last most important thing to consider is this: eat real food. Following the keto diet requires more meal planning and more food preparation, but it is well worth it in the long run. And following the keto diet does not mean you have to give up good food or treats. There are endless recipes for meals and snack, even dessert type snack that will keep your food intake within the keto requirements and keep you feeling full and satisfied. Don't be afraid to explore different menus, recipes, and options. You may be surprised at how flexible keto living really is.

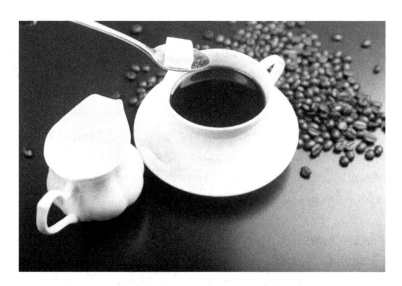

# Conclusion

Thank you for making it through to the end of *Intermittent Fasting: Ketogenic Diet for Maximum Weight Loss*, let's hope it was informative and able to provide you with all of the tools you need to achieve your goals whatever they may be. I hope that this book provided you with all the knowledge you need to begin your journey into the wonderful world of ketogenic dieting and intermittent fasting.

The next step is to take advantage of the knowledge you have learned from reading this book and plan the first day of the rest of your life. As we said, the keto diet and intermittent fasting is a lifestyle change, one that will change your life and the way you look at food forever. We have given you an in-depth understanding of how the keto diet works and how intermittent fasting fits into your particular lifestyle. We have discussed the history of keto dieting and intermittent fasting. We have looked at good and bad foods and discussed how to make recipes and meal plans that work for you.

Finally, if you found this book useful in any way, a review on Amazon is always appreciated!

# Addendum

## Recipes for Beginners

Keto recipes do not need to be difficult. Many are very easy compilations of a few simple foods. Some recipes are more complicated. Anywhere you look you will find samples of both. It is very important that you select menu plans and recipes that fit into your lifestyle. If your day is short on time, you may not be able to finish a complicated recipe. Many followers of the keto lifestyle find it is easier to do much of their meal planning on their days off work, sometimes cooking a week's worth of meat, eggs, muffins, et cetera to use throughout the week. We have gathered some sample recipes here to assist you with beginning your new lifestyle. The recipes have been divided into breakfast, lunch, dinner, sides, snacks, and appetizers.

# Breakfast Recipes

## *Keto Pancakes*

Gather the following ingredients:

Eggs, four large
Softened cream cheese, four ounces
Almond flour, .5 Cup
Lemon zest, one teaspoon (optional for flavor)

Always use real butter for frying and serving

After all the ingredients are combined fully, set a medium to large sized skillet over medium heat and melt one or two tablespoons of butter in it. Then add three to five tablespoons of batter (depending on the desired size), flip pancake when bubbles form all over the top side, serve with more real butter. No Syrup!

## *Smooth Fruit Smoothie*

In a blender, combine the following ingredients:

Coconut milk, one to two cups
Frozen blackberries, one to two cups
Frozen raspberries, one to two cups
Frozen strawberries, one to two cups
Baby spinach, .5 to one cup

Optional—use frozen berries or shredded coconut for a pretty garnish

Depending on whether you are making this for one person or two people will determine the measurement you use. The first measurement is for one serving, and the second measurement is for two people. Mix well, pour the smoothie into a glass, garnish as desired, and enjoy!

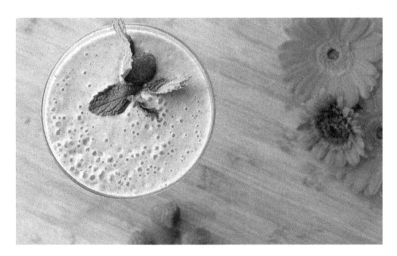

## *Blueberry Muffins Keto Style*

Mix well in a large bowl the following ingredients:

Almond milk, unsweetened, .34 cup
Almond flour, 2.5 cups
Keto friendly sugar, .34 cup
Eggs, 3 large
Baking soda, one-half of one teaspoon
Kosher salt, .5 teaspoon
Baking powder, one and one-half teaspoons
Melted butter, .34 cup
Vanilla extract, one teaspoon
Fresh (not frozen) blueberries (or strawberries, blackberries, or raspberries), .5 cup

Preheat oven to 350 degrees and set oven rack in the middle of the oven. Mix all the ingredients together except the blueberries. When all the other ingredients are mixed well, add the blueberries (or other fruit) and gently fold the berries into the batter. Prepare a twelve-cup muffin tin with paper cups. Spoon equal amounts of the batter into each of the twelve cups. Bake the muffins on the center oven rack for a total of twenty-five minutes. Check for doneness by inserting a toothpick. If it comes out clean, the muffins are done cooking.

Eggs in Pepper Rings

Gather the following ingredients:

Eggs, three to four
Pepper rings, green, yellow, or red as desired, sliced into .5-inch-thick rings

In a large skillet over medium heat melt two tablespoons of butter. Add three to four green pepper rings, cooking them two to three minutes on the first side. Flip the rings over and crack a raw egg into each ring. Season each egg with the desired amount of kosher salt, pepper, oregano, or parsley—season to your personal taste! Cook the eggs from two to four minutes to your personal taste. Serve and enjoy.

## *Hash with Brussel Sprouts*

Gather the following ingredients:

One-inch pieces of bacon, six strips total
Onion, .5 cup chopped
Brussel Sprouts, one cup trimmed and chopped
Black pepper, red pepper, and salt, .25 teaspoon each
Water, three tablespoons
Fresh garlic, two minced cloves
Eggs, four large

Fry the bacon in a large skillet over medium heat, removing the bacon from the skillet when it is crispy and placing it on a draining rack or paper-towel covered plate. Break the bacon into one-inch pieces. Leaving accumulated bacon fat in the skillet, add the onion, garlic, and Brussel sprouts, sautéing until the sprouts are tender. Use a spoon to make four wells in the mixture, deep enough to reach the bottom of the skillet. Crack one egg into each well, then use salt and pepper to season the entire pan of hash. Cook eggs two to five minutes, to desired doneness, then sprinkle with bacon pieces and serve.

## *Avocado Bacon Balls*

Gather all ingredients:

Avocados, four
Cream cheese, one block (not all will be used)
Bacon, raw, four to eight slices

Heat the broiler section of the oven and line a small baking sheet with aluminum foil. Peel all four avocados, cutting them in half lengthwise, and remove and discard the pits. Fill one half of each avocado with cream cheese and place the two halves back together. Wrap each avocado with bacon to completely cover the avocado and secure the loose end of the bacon with a toothpick. Place the bacon-covered avocados on the foil-lined baking sheet and broil, five minutes on each side, until the bacon is crispy. Serve immediately.

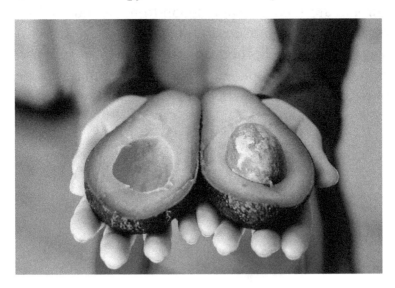

## *Easy Breakfast Stacks*

Gather all ingredients:

Breakfast sausage patties, three
Avocado, one mashed
Black pepper and kosher salt
Eggs, three large

Chives for garnish and mild to hot sauce as desired

Mash avocado and set aside. Cook the sausage patties, following the directions on the box. Place a large skillet over medium heat and melt three tablespoons of butter. Break the eggs into the skillet, season as desired, and cook two to five minutes to the desired doneness. Place a sausage patty on the plate, spoon mashed avocado on top, then lay the cooked egg over the avocado. Garnish top of egg with chives or sprinkle on a little hot sauce as you prefer.

## *Toasted Cauliflower*

Gather all ingredients:

Cauliflower, one medium head gently shredded
Egg, one large
Cheddar cheese, one cup shredded
Pepper, salt, and garlic powder, .5 teaspoon each

After preheating the oven to 425 degrees, set the oven rack in the middle. Line a baking sheet with aluminum foil or parchment paper. After gently shredding the cauliflower place it in a bowl and microwave on high for eight minutes. Thoroughly drain the cauliflower, using paper towels or a fine strainer or cheesecloth, until it's dry.

Add the seasonings, eggs, and cheddar cheese to the cauliflower mixture in the bowl. Mix all ingredients thoroughly. Spoon the mixture onto a buttered cookie sheet in round or square shapes roughly the size of a slice of bread, about one-quarter inch thick. Bake shapes eighteen to twenty minutes until the shapes are golden brown. Eat plain or top with any desired topping like a fried egg, tomato slices, or mashed avocado.

## *Bacon (or Sausage) and Eggs*

Gather all ingredients:

Eggs, two per person
Bacon (or sausage) two to three pieces per person

Fry the bacon to the desired doneness. If using sausage then follow directions on the package. Leave some of the bacon or sausage grease in the skillet to use for cooking the eggs—either scrambled or fried as you prefer. If no grease is left over from cooking the meat, then add two tablespoons of butter to the skillet. Season the eggs with salt and pepper as desired. Serve and enjoy!

## *Bulletproof Coffee (Perfect for Morning of Fasting)*

Combine one cup of hot, freshly brewed black coffee, one to two tablespoons of coconut oil, and one to two tablespoons of unsalted butter in a blender. Blend on high until well blended. Drink immediately.

# Lunch Recipes

(These can also be used as dinner recipes)

## *Easy meatballs*

Gather all ingredients:

Ground beef, one pound
Salt, .25 teaspoon
Pepper, .25 teaspoon
Red pepper, .25 teaspoon
Chives, chopped, one teaspoon

Mix all ingredients together in a bowl. Roll all this meat mixture into round shapes about the size of golf balls. Line a baking sheet with aluminum foil or parchment paper. Bake the meatballs at 400 degrees for fifteen minutes. Freeze extras for quick meals later.

## *Philly Cheesesteak Roll-Up*

Gather all ingredients:

Shredded beef, four ounces
Shredded provolone cheese, four ounces
Chopped onion and green pepper as desired, one tablespoon each
Low-carb flour tortillas (available in the bread section of most large stores)
Oil, olive or canola, two tablespoons
Salt and pepper, .25 teaspoon each

Place a large skillet over medium heat and warm the olive oil. Add the beef to the pan. As soon as the meat is completely browned, drain it and return it to the skillet. If you are using the peppers and/or onions, add them to the skillet and cook until these are slightly soft. Spoon mixture into center of tortilla and top with shredded cheese. Fold over or roll burrito style and enjoy.

## *Turkey Wraps with Ranch Dressing*

Gather all ingredients:

Leaf lettuce, two to three leaves, washed and patted dry
Turkey or ham, four to six slices
Cheese, sliced, any flavor, two to three slices
Onion, sliced thinly
Green pepper, sliced thinly

Place one washed leaf lettuce on a plate. Add layers of turkey or ham, sliced cheese, sliced onion or bell pepper, and salt and pepper to taste. Drizzle with ranch dressing or oil and vinegar. Roll and enjoy.

## *Chicken Thighs with Cabbage and Cheese*

Gather all ingredients:

Chicken thighs, four
Olive oil, .25 cup
Salt and pepper to taste
Cheddar cheese, shredded, .5 cup
Cabbage, chopped

Coat the four chicken thighs with olive oil and season with salt and pepper to taste. Bake 1 hour in a covered baking dish, remove from oven, and top with shredded cheddar cheese. Serve on a bed of chopped cabbage.

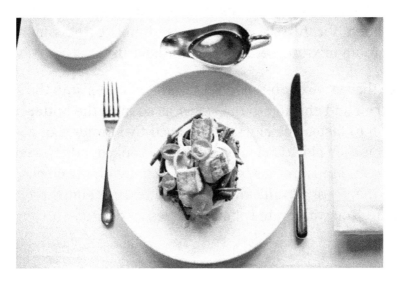

## *Mushroom Chicken*

Gather all ingredients:

Chicken breast, two flattened and tenderized
Onion, one small
Mushrooms, .5 cup canned or fresh
Salt, .5 teaspoon
Thyme, .5 teaspoon
Butter, three tablespoons unsalted
Coconut milk, .3 cup

Slice mushrooms and onion into thin slices. Place a large skillet over medium heat and melt one tablespoon of butter. Gently place the onions and mushrooms to the skillet and stir gently and often for five to six minutes. Remove the onion and mushroom mixture, setting aside for later use.

Place the last two tablespoons of unsalted butter into the skillet and then add chicken to the skillet as soon as the butter melts. Season to taste. The chicken will need five minutes of cooking time on each side. Once the chicken is cooked, add the cooked onions and mushrooms back to the skillet with the chicken and pour the coconut milk over all. Let mixture simmer for one minute. Top with grated cheddar cheese if desired

## *Shrimp Salad*

Gather all ingredients:

Shrimp, frozen peeled and deveined, one cup
Tomatoes, cherry, .5 cup
Lettuce, torn into bite-sized pieces, one cup
Butter, two tablespoons

Thaw and rinse one cup of small peeled and deveined shrimp according to the package instructions. Dry the shrimp by patting it with a paper towel. Cook the shrimp in a skillet in two tablespoons of melted butter over medium heat until done. Shrimp will turn pink when it is done. Serve over a bed of mixed greens and cherry tomatoes.

## *Keto Chili*

Gather all ingredients:

Ground beef, one pound
Onion, finely chopped, .25 cup
Pepper, green, chopped, .25 cup
Chili mix, any brand, one packet

Brown one pound of ground beef (no need to go lean, fatter is better) in a skillet over medium heat. Drain the ground beef and rinse after cooking. Return ground beef to skillet. Add the onion and the green pepper. Add chili powder mix according to directions on the package. Mix well, simmer for fifteen to twenty minutes over medium heat, and serve with a generous dollop of sour cream if desired.

## *Tuna Wraps*

Gather all ingredients:

Tuna, one can, in oil, drained well
Lettuce, iceberg, shredded, .5 cup
Lettuce, leaf, two to three leaves
Cheese, Swiss, two tablespoons

Mix drained tuna, shredded iceberg lettuce, and Swiss cheese in a bowl. Spoon desired amount of the mixture onto leaf lettuce, roll, and enjoy.

## *Mushroom Swiss Burger*

Gather all ingredients:

Ground beef, formed into patty, .5 cup
Mushroom, button, small can
Cheese, Swiss, two slices
Sour cream

Cook one hamburger patty thoroughly until done, season as desired. Warm one small can of button mushroom in a pan over medium heat. Top the cooked burger with sliced Swiss cheese and a mound of warm button mushrooms. Sour cream can be used as a garnish if desired. A mixed lettuce salad will complete the meal.

## *Chicken Salad*

Gather all ingredients:

Chicken breast, one pound
Celery, three ribs diced
Mayonnaise, .5 cup
Mustard, brown, two tablespoons
Salt, .5 teaspoon
Chopped dill, fresh, two tablespoons
Pecans, .25 cup chopped

Boil the chicken breast until it is cooked thoroughly, about thirty minutes. Set the chicken aside to cool. When the chicken is cool cut the breast into bite-sized pieces. After placing the cubed chicken in a bowl add the other ingredients. Combine all ingredients thoroughly until the chicken is fully coated. Cover and refrigerate one hour until cold. Serve cold with keto friendly crackers or tortillas.

# Dinner Recipes

(These can also be used as lunch recipes, especially during a long, lazy weekend)

## *Bowl of Egg Roll*

Gather all ingredients:

Olive oil, one tablespoon plus one tablespoon
Beef, ground, one pound
Cabbage, five cups shredded
Chicken broth, .25 cup
Ginger, minced, .5 tablespoon
Carrots, one cup shredded
Onion, one cup chopped
Garlic, three cloves crushed
Soy sauce, two tablespoons
Vinegar, apple cider, two tablespoons
Salt and pepper, .5 teaspoon each
Sesame oil, one teaspoon

Place a large skillet over medium heat and add one tablespoon of olive oil. Add the ground beef to the skillet as soon as the oil is warm and stirring often until it is fully cooked. Rinse and drain the beef and save for later use.

Place the remaining olive oil in the skillet, adding the garlic, ginger, carrots, and onions. Sauté this mixture for two to three minutes.

Return the cooked ground beef to the skillet and mix well with the veggie mixture. Pour the chicken broth over the mixture in the skillet, scraping the bottom of the pan to get all the glazing off. Add the soy sauce, salt, pepper, vinegar, and cabbage. Cover the skillet and simmer on medium heat for fifteen minutes, or just until the cabbage feels done to your desired taste/texture. Serve in a bowl with a drizzle of soy sauce on top.

## *Baked Pork Loin with Loaded Broccoli*

Gather all ingredients:

Pork loin, two pounds
Broccoli, florets, one cup
Water, three tablespoons
Cheese, shredded cheddar, two tablespoons
Onions, chopped, two tablespoons
Sour cream or cream cheese if desired

In a 400-degree oven on a middle oven rack bake a two-pound pork loin for twenty minutes per pound, or until the loin reaches an internal temperature of 145 degrees. Remove the pork loin from the oven at the end of the cooking period. While the pork loin is resting add one cup of broccoli florets to a microwave safe bowl, adding three tablespoons of water, cover the bowl firmly with plastic wrap, and microwave on high for three minutes. Drain any remaining liquid; top the florets with the shredded cheese and the onions. Place the florets on a plate and top with generous dollops of sour cream or cream cheese. Slice the pork loin to accompany.

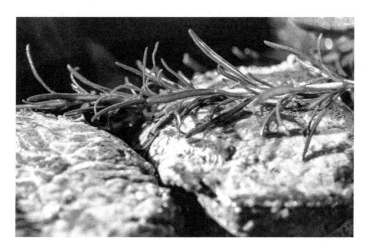

## *Chicken Breast Supreme*

Gather all ingredients:

Chicken breast, one per person
Cream cheese, two tablespoons per chicken breast
Green onion, one tablespoon finely chopped per chicken breast
Bacon, two pieces per chicken breast

Preheat the oven to 375 degrees and set the oven rack in the middle of the oven. Wrap one chicken breast in plastic wrap and pound it out to about one-fourth inch thickness. Uncover the chicken breast. Mix together two tablespoons of cream cheese with one tablespoon of the chopped green onion. Spread this mixture over one side of the chicken breast. Gently roll the chicken breast into a tube shape to hide the cream cheese. Wrap two slices of bacon around each rolled chicken breast and secure with a toothpick. Place the rolled breasts on a foil-lined baking sheet and bake for thirty minutes. Serve with a salad of mixed lettuce.

## *Fish Sticks*

Gather all ingredients:

Fish, cod or whitefish, cut into .5-inch strips
Egg, two, well beaten
Cheese, parmesan, grated, one cup
Pork rinds, crushed, two cups

Preheat oven to 400 degrees. Dip strips of codfish or whitefish in the beaten egg and roll in a mixture of the grated parmesan cheese and crushed pork rinds. After ten minutes in a 350-degree oven turn the sticks and cook for an additional ten minutes. These are best served with mixed salad or slaw.

## *Grilled Kebobs*

Cube steak or chicken breast and spear on a kabob, alternating with pearl onion, button mushrooms, and cherry tomatoes. Grill over coals or propane outside for twenty minutes or bake in a 350-degree oven on a foil lined cookie sheet for twenty minutes.

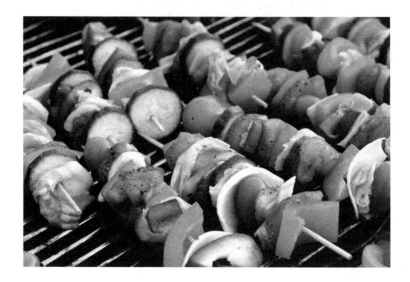

## Chicken Fried Cauliflower Rice

Gather all ingredients:

Cauliflower, one medium sized head with stem removed
Chicken breast, two, cooked, diced, and chilled
Canola oil, three teaspoons
Scallions, .25 cup thinly sliced
Mixed peas and carrots, one cup
Eggs, two large lightly beaten
Garlic, three cloves minced
Fresh ginger, one one-inch long piece, grated
Soy sauce, .25 cup
Sesame oil, two tablespoons

After cutting the cauliflower into chunks, use a food processor to pulse the cauliflower, in small batches, until it is coarse in texture like rice. If no food processor is available, the cauliflower can be finely chopped with a sharp knife.

Using a wok or placing large skillet over medium heat, place one tablespoon of canola oil. When the oil has warmed, place the eggs in the pan and scramble them quickly. Set the eggs aside in a bowl for use later. Add the remaining two tablespoons oil into the wok or skillet and warm. Place ginger and garlic in the pan. Cook this mixture while stirring constantly for about one minute. Add the peas, carrots, scallions, and cauliflower to the skillet, stirring often until the vegetables are tender, about ten minutes.

During the time the vegetables are cooking, stir the soy sauce and sesame oil together in a small bowl. Stir this sauce and the chicken into the cauliflower mixture. Cook this mixture for five minutes. Then pour the eggs back to the skillet.

## *Italian Meatballs*

Gather all ingredients:

Ground pork or turkey, .5 pound
Ground beef, .5 pound
Cream, heavy, .25 cup
Parmesan cheese, grated, .25 cup
Egg, one large beaten
Salt and pepper, .25 teaspoon each
Parsley flakes, one teaspoon
Garlic, one small clove chopped finely
Onion, one tablespoon finely chopped

After placing the rack in the middle of the oven, preheat to 400 degrees. Thoroughly mix beef and pork in medium-sized bowl. Add all the remaining ingredients to the meat mixture and mix well by hand. Divide the mixture into twelve evenly sized portions and roll these portions into meatballs.

Place the meatballs on a foil-lined baking sheet, with space in between. Bake the meatballs for twenty minutes. When serving, top with shredded mozzarella cheese and bits of chopped parsley.

## *Creamy Kale Chicken Bake*

Gather all ingredients:

Chicken breast, cooked and cubed, three cups
Kale, two cups raw
Red onion, two tablespoons diced
Cream cheese, softened, eighteen ounces
Mozzarella cheese, shredded,.75 cup
Parmesan cheese, .25 cup, shredded
Butter, one tablespoon unsalted
Mayonnaise, .35 cup
Sour cream, .5 cup
Salt and pepper, .25 teaspoon each
Garlic powder, .25 teaspoon

After placing the oven rack in the middle of the oven, preheat to 400 degrees.

Place butter to melt in a large skillet using medium heat. Add onion and stir until it is see-through, about two to three minutes, stirring often. Add the kale and sauté with the onion until the kale wilts. Season this mixture with salt and pepper.

Mix the sour cream, mayonnaise, garlic powder, and cream cheese in a bowl, mixing all ingredients until smooth. Place this mixture with the kale in the skillet. After mixing all, then add the cubed chicken and the mozzarella cheese and mix well. Pour contents of the skillet into a buttered eight-by-eight baking dish.

Top with parmesan cheese and bake uncovered for twenty minutes. If desired, serve over shredded uncooked cabbage or shredded zucchini to mimic noodles.

## *Three Cheese Chicken*

Gather all ingredients:

Chicken breast, three to four
Parmesan cheese, .5 cup
Swiss cheese, one cup
Cheddar cheese, one cup

This meal is deceptively simple. Butter and season the chicken breasts and bake for forty-five minutes in a baking dish in a 400-degree oven. Remove the dish from oven, cover with all three cheeses. Bake an additional fifteen minutes. Serve with steamed asparagus.

## *Grilled Rosemary Pork Chops*

Gather all ingredients:

Pork chops, four loin chops, bone-in or boneless
Butter, one stick
Olive oil, one tablespoon melted
Garlic, two cloves minced
Salt and pepper, .5 teaspoon each
Rosemary, one tablespoon chopped

After placing the oven rack in the middle preheat the oven to 375 degrees. Mix together the melted butter, rosemary, garlic and save for later use.

Sprinkle the salt and pepper on the pork chops. Using a large skillet over medium heat, warm the olive oil. Add the pork chops and sear until golden, four minutes on each side. Remove the pork chops from the skillet and place in an oven-safe baking dish. Brush chops generously with garlic butter mixture and bake uncovered for fifteen minutes.

## Appetizers

### *Deviled Eggs*

Gather all ingredients:

Eggs, six
Salt and pepper, .25 teaspoon each
Mayonnaise, one tablespoon
Mustard, one teaspoon
Paprika, powdered

Peel six hard-boiled eggs and cut in half down the long side of the egg. Pop the yolks out, placing them in a bowl for mashing. Add salt and pepper to mashed yolks. Pour in the mustard and the mayonnaise, mix well and scoop the mashed yolks onto the egg whites. Use the powdered paprika to sprinkle over the top of the yolk if desired.

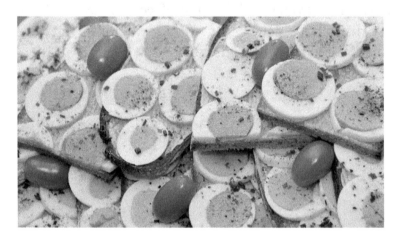

## *Bacon Wrapped Brussel Sprouts*

Gather all ingredients:

Brussel sprouts, twelve large
Bacon, raw, 12 slices
Pepper, .25 teaspoon
Sour cream

Wrap each of twelve large Brussel sprouts with one strip of bacon. Sprinkle pepper over the sprouts. The oven should be heated to 375 degrees. Use aluminum foil to line a baking sheet. Place bacon wrapped Brussel sprouts on the foil covered baking sheet. In 30 minutes remove them from the oven. Sour cream makes a great dipping sauce.

## *Pickle Bacon Wraps*

Gather all ingredients:

Pickle spears, twelve
Bacon, sliced, raw, 12 slices
Ranch dressing

Wrap pickle spears with sliced bacon and secure with a toothpick. Place the bacon-wrapped spears on a foil covered baking sheet and bake for twenty-five minutes in a 425-degree oven. Serve with ranch dressing for dipping.

## Baked Shrimp

Gather all ingredients:

Shrimp, eight medium size, raw
Olive oil, one tablespoon
Egg, one, beaten
Coconut flour, .5 teaspoon
Coconut, three tablespoons, unsweetened, shredded

In a bowl combine the shredded coconut and the coconut flour. Dip shrimp, one at a time, into beaten egg, then roll in shredded coconut/coconut flour mixture. Line a baking pan with aluminum foil and place the fish sticks evenly spaced on it, baking at 300 degrees, twenty minutes per side.

## Chicken Tenders

Gather all ingredients:

Chicken breast, one pound, cut in strips
Egg, one large
Heavy whipping cream, one tablespoon
Almond flour, one cup
Salt and pepper, .25 teaspoon each

Season the chicken strips with the salt and pepper. Dip each strip into egg beaten with one tablespoon of the heavy cream, then dip into the almond flour. Line a baking sheet with aluminum foil and place the tenders on it, evenly spaced, baking for thirty minutes in a 350-degree oven. Dip tenders in your choice of ranch dressing or sour cream.

## *Salami Rolls*

Gather all ingredients:

Salami, one pound, thin sliced
Pepper, green or yellow, thinly sliced
Cream cheese, one pound at room temperature

After laying one large piece of plastic wrap on the counter, lightly spread the cream cheese on the plastic wrap, and covering it with another piece of plastic wrap. Use a rolling pin to flatten the cream cheese to a thin layer, about .25 inches thick. Do not let the cream cheese go beyond the edge of the plastic wrap. After removing the top layer of plastic wrap, lay the green pepper slices over the cream cheese, then add the salami slices. Replace the top layer of wrap and turn the whole thing over, putting the salami on the bottom and the cream cheese layer is on top. Take off the layer of plastic that is now on top, using the bottom sheet to roll the salami into a log. Once it is fully rolled slice the log into thin slices.

## *Fried Avocado Slices*

Gather all ingredients:

Avocados, three
Oil, canola or olive, one cup
Flour, almond, 1.5 cups
Egg, one
Salt and pepper, .25 teaspoon each
Ranch dressing or sour cream

Beat egg in a medium sized bowl. In another bowl, mix the flour with the salt and pepper. Peel each avocado, slice lengthwise and remove the seed. Slice each half into vertical slices about one-half inch thick. Coat each slice of avocado in the egg mixture, and then dip into the almond flour until well coated. Warm the oil over medium heat in a large skillet. When the oil warms, carefully add avocado strips, cooking for no more than one minute or until the strips are a light brown color. Serve with ranch dressing or sour cream for dipping.

## *Chicken Nuggets*

Gather all ingredients:

Chicken breast, one pound, tenders
Butter, three to four tablespoons
Coconut flour, three tablespoons
Paprika, one teaspoon
Onion powder, one teaspoon
Black pepper, .5 teaspoon
Garlic powder, one teaspoon
Salt, one teaspoon

Mix all seasoning into flour in a bowl. Add tenders to flour mixture and coat well. Melt the butter over medium heat in a large skillet. Add the chicken tenders to the melted butter. Fry for ten minutes on each side. Serve with celery sticks and ranch dressing.

## *Cucumber Sausage Bites with Cream Cheese*

Gather all ingredients:

Summer sausage, one logs
Cucumber, one medium
Cream cheese, one brick
Green onion, three chopped finely

Use an electric mixer to mix the onions and cream cheese in a bowl. Slice the sausage and the cucumber into one-quarter inch thick slices. Place the sausage on a tray, the top with a slice of cucumber. Pipe cream cheese on top of the cucumber slices with a pastry bag.

## *Sampler Platter*

Gather all ingredients:

Salami, one log
Ham steak
Cheddar cheese, block
Swiss cheese, block
Olives, green and black
Pickles, baby dills
Cucumber, whole
Celery, one bunch
Peppers, green and red

Slice the salami into one-quarter inch thick slices, do the same with the cucumber. Cut the ham steak and both cheeses into bite-size squares. Drain the olives and the pickles. Cut the end off the celery and slice into sticks. Arrange all items on a platter or wooden bowl and serve with low-carb crackers.

# Sides

## *Mashed cauliflower*

Bake or steam one head of cauliflower broken into pieces. Add butter and salt and mash like a potato.

## *Loaded broccoli*

Steam or bake one bunch of broccolis separated into florets. Garnish with shredded cheddar cheese, bacon bits, and sour cream.

## *Roasted cabbage*

Cut one-half head of cabbage into four wedges. Brush olive oil on each wedge and sprinkle with pepper and salt. Bake for thirty minutes in a 450-degree oven.

## *Button mushroom*

Melt two tablespoons of butter in a medium saucepan using medium heat. Add two cups of sliced fresh mushrooms and stir until soft.

## *Cheesy Creamed Spinach*

Gather all ingredients:

Salt and pepper, .25 teaspoon each
Parmesan cheese, .5 cup
Cream, one cup, heavy
Cream cheese, four ounces
Butter, one tablespoon
Butter, three tablespoons
Onion powder, one teaspoon
Garlic, two cloves minced
Spinach, two ten-ounce packages frozen and thawed or fresh

Sauté the onion and garlic in three tablespoons of butter over medium heat in a medium skillet. Add the spinach, cover and cook on low, five minutes. In another pot mix the cream cheese, parmesan cheese, heavy cream, and one tablespoon of butter. Cook these on medium until the cream cheese is melted, then whisk until all ingredients are smooth. After adding the salt and pepper, cover the spinach mixture with the melted cheese.

## *Cole Slaw*

Gather all ingredients:

Cabbage, green, one head
Salt and pepper, .25 teaspoon each
Mayonnaise, one cup

Using a food processor, sharp knife, or mandolin slicer, shred the cabbage. Put the cabbage in a bowl and add the mayo, salt, and pepper. Stir well. Let slaw sit for ten to fifteen minutes before serving.

## Cold Mixed Veggies

In a large bowl combine chunk of cauliflower, broccoli florets, and mushroom slices. Toss lightly with oil and vinegar dressing.

## Turnip Fries

Trim the ends off four medium-sized turnips and cut them into wedges. Brush the wedges with olive oil and a mixture of .25 teaspoon each of salt, pepper, and garlic powder. Cover a baking sheet with aluminum foil and bake the turnip wedges at 400 degrees for forty minutes, twenty minutes per side.

## Roasted Radishes

Trim the ends and tops off two bunches of radishes. In a small bowl mix .5 cup of olive oil, .25 cup of lemon juice, and .25 teaspoon each of pepper and salt. Cover the radishes with this sauce and mix well. Bake radishes for thirty minutes in a 400-degree oven on a baking sheet lined with aluminum foil.

## Easy Garlic and Bacon Green Beans

Using fresh or canned green beans, place them in a casserole dish. Add one clove of garlic, minced, and one-half cup of bacon bits. Bake for fifteen minutes in a 350-degree oven.

## Keto Snacks

Snacking is not recommended on the keto diet. All needed calories should come from well-balanced meals. However, there are times when hunger distracts us, and we can't think about anything but our growling tummies. Following is a list of ten of the best keto-friendly snacks, guaranteed to take the edge off the biggest hunger.

- Hard-boiled eggs

- Cheddar cheese wedges

- Beef jerky

- Pork rinds

- Avocado slices

- Green olives

- Dill pickle wedges

- Celery sticks

- Mozzarella string cheese

- Dark chocolate

**Extra Bonus:**

# Exercises to Help Maximize Weight Loss

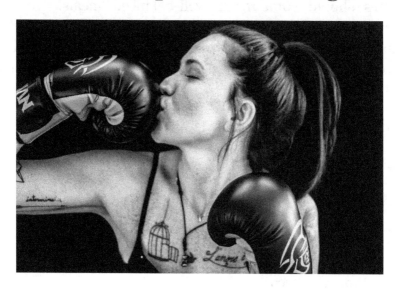

Whenever one begins a new diet, there is a period of adjustment to the new eating plan. One thing many people worry about is losing muscle tone. This is not as big a consideration on the keto diet since the keto diet is designed to eliminate fatty waste from the body while maintaining good cellular growth. As with any diet, weight loss on the keto diet will be aided with the addition of exercise. Don't panic. I'm not suggesting you immediately begin training for a marathon, although you might eventually feel so good that you want to! But I do want to show you how incorporating some movement into your daily routine can help you with your weight loss goals.

The easiest method of exercising is walking. Man was built to walk. Our bodies crave the type of movement that walking gives us. Long strides accompanied by loose arm swings—perfection! Walking is fairly simple, too. It requires no special equipment other than a comfortable pair of walking shoes.

If you have access to a pool, then swimming is another marvelous form of exercise. Whether you are swimming laps of merely walking through the water, you will burn calories.

Keep in mind that any physical movement can be considered exercise. Anything that gets your body moving will help you burn more calories and fat and push you that much closer to your weight loss success. Walk the dog, push a lawnmower around the yard, throw the football with the kids, roller skate, play volleyball or basketball, jump rope, rake leaves—in other words, get out and move. Moving is exercise, and exercise doesn't need to be boring.

Don't overlook weight lifting. I'm not talking about the heavy dumbbell lift guaranteed to make you look like Popeye. There are two ways to lift weights. Smaller weights lifted at a higher number of repetitions will lead to lean muscles. Heavier weights lifted until the muscle is fatigued will result in muscle mass growth. Both methods are desirable for building that strong, lean body you are striving for.

Boxing is another good aerobic and strength combining exercise you can use to facilitate weight loss. Again, you don't really need to purchase any special equipment. While it would be nice to have a workout bag hanging in the basement for you to pummel, you can get the same effect by punching a pillow or the dancing around punching the air. The key is to keep moving.

If you feel the need to have specific exercises to help you on your journey, that's easy enough. There is any number of sources for exercise. Some of the more popular ones you can do at home are squats, lunges, pushups, planks, and jumping jacks.

It is not necessary to join a gym unless you really want to or you find you need the motivation of a personal trainer to reach your goals. Don't overlook the local community college or recreation center. Many of them offer exercise classes or informal sports teams. Any of these things will get you moving. And moving is exercise.

CPSIA information can be obtained
at www.ICGtesting.com
Printed in the USA
BVHW041721121120
593183BV00007B/536